Kate Gould

5th February 1977 – 9th October 2017

From a collection of books gathered by Kate Gould for her PhD on the ways in which media coverage of "pink Viagra" represented and constructed female sexuality; in her years at the front line of gender politics as part of the global sisterhood; and as a passionate campaigner for the truth and rights of women.

<u>Critical Sisters posted this on hearing of Kate's death:</u>

'Love and anger course through the radical feminist community compelling each of us to question, debate and create change. Many of us never met Kate in real life, and yet she spoke our truth often in the face of hostility. Her clear and unwavering voice rang out through her writing - righteous, powerful and insightful. Without ego and free from artifice - Kate's bravery, shining intellect and warmth have inspired many of us. Kate gave to each of us; and her memory and work continue to give us strength. We will miss our sister.'

ALSO BY MARISA ACOCELLA MARCHETTO

JUST WHO THE HELL IS SHE, ANYWAY?

CANCER VIXEN

CHEMO#1. AUGUST 12, 2004. I APPLIED *VIVA GLAM* LIPGLASS BY M.A.C.

CancerVixen

A TRUE STORY

Marisa Acocella Marchetto

FOURTH ESTATE • London

First published in Great Britain in 2007 by
Fourth Estate
An imprint of HarperCollins*Publishers*
77–85 Fulham Palace Road
London W6 8JB
www.4thestate.co.uk

1 3 5 7 9 8 6 4 2

A catalogue record for this book is
available from the British Library

ISBN-10 0-00-722163-0
ISBN-13 978-0-00-722163-9

Out of concern for the privacy of individuals depicted here,
the author has changed the names of certain individuals, as well
as potentially identifying descriptive details concerning them.

Manufactured in Singapore

FOR SILVANO

WHAT HAPPENS WHEN A SHOE-CRAZY, LIPSTICK-OBSESSED, WINE-SWILLING, PASTA-SLURPING, FASHION-FANATIC, SINGLE-FOREVER, ABOUT-TO-GET-MARRIED BIG-CITY GIRL CARTOONIST (ME, MARISA ACOCELLA) WITH A FABULOUS LIFE FINDS...

A LUMP IN HER BREAST?!?

HERE IS THE TUMOR, IT LOOKS LIKE A BLACK HOLE

I NOTICED SOMETHING FISHY WHILE SWIMMING IN APRIL.

WHY DOES MY ARM HURT?

ON MY WAY OUT, I HEARD THAT STUPID *KANSAS* SONG IN MY HEAD...

...ALL WE ARE IS DUST IN THE--

-- OH SHUT UP.

5 MINUTES LATER...

HEY BOB, I KNOW YOU'RE ON DEADLINE FOR THE *TIMES*, BUT I HAVE GOOD DIRT FOR YOU... I HEARD THAT THE FORMERLY ON FIRE *LIT* CHICK IS SO DESPERATE FOR PRESS, SHE'S CALLING IN ITEMS ABOUT *HERSELF*.

WHO CARES? TALK TO ME ABOUT SOMETHING SERIOUS!

MY BEST FRIEND FOREVER (THAT'S "BFF") BOB

OK, I'M ON MY WAY TO A BREAST SPECIALIST BECAUSE OF A LUMP...

...BOB...?

...HELLO..?!

HEY... YOU WERE THE ONE WHO WANTED "SERIOUS"!

LATER, IN BREAST SPECIALIST DR. CHRISTOPHER MILLS'S OFFICE...

WHY ARE YOU HERE *ALONE*?

THIS JUST HAPPENED AN HOUR AND A HALF AGO!

GOWN #2

WHEN A DOCTOR CARES ABOUT YOUR COMFORT, IT'S A SIGN HE'S A GOOD ONE.

AND THEN I FIND OUT THAT HE ISN'T *JUST* A BREAST SPECIALIST, DR. MILLS IS A BREAST *SURGEON*.

A KNIVES
CUT
BLOOD
INCISION
SURGERY
SURGEON.
(SO MUCH FOR MY COMFORT.)

4

WHEN I GOT HOME, I CALLED MY STELLAR SUPPORT GROUP, STARTING WITH MY MOM.

ARE YOU SITTING?

MY MOTHER, AKA "(S)MOTHER," ALL BIG HAIR, BIG JEWELRY, AND BIG BIG BIG PERSONALITY, SHE'S THE NEW JERSEY VERSION OF SOPHIA LOREN.

MY THROAT'S SORE, MY KNEES HURT, THANKS FOR ASKING, WHY...

WHAT'S THE MATTER?

OK, *NOW* I'M SITTING.

SLAM!

LA TOILETTE

THIS IS ALL *YOUR* FAULT... I TOLD YOU TO GET THE NEGATIVITY OUT OF YOUR LIFE!

AND YOU BETTER NOT DRAW ME ON THE THRONE!

DON'T LISTEN TO YOUR MOTHER.

← KIMBERLEY, MY BFF AND MARRIED MOTHER OF TWO IN CONNECTICUT

WHERE YOU'LL ALWAYS FIND ME, AT MY DRAWING BOARD →

MAREESE... IT'S PROBABLY JUST FIBROIDS.

↙ SHARON, MY BFF AND HAIRCOLORIST TO THE STARS

RELAX... YOU'VE BEEN HAVING MAMMOGRAMS, RIGHT?

← ANNIE, MY BFF AND FASHION EXECUTRIX

I'VE NEVER HAD A MAMMOGRAM.

YOU'VE *NEVER* HAD A MAMMOGRAM?! I'M GOING TO KILL YOU!

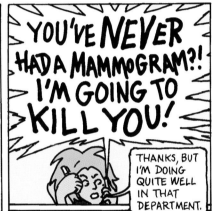

THANKS, BUT I'M DOING QUITE WELL IN THAT DEPARTMENT.

LISTEN CANCER, YA SICK BASTARD...

...FINALLY, AT 43, I'M GETTING MARRIED FOR THE FIRST TIME...

I want a dress that's simple and white and kinda tight.

...AND DAVID REMNICK, EDITOR IN CHIEF OF *THE NEW YORKER*, WANTS TO PUBLISH MORE OF MY CARTOONS...

OK, I'LL DOUBLE MY EFFORT.

...NOW IS *NOT* A GOOD TIME!

THAT NIGHT, SILVANO RANG ME FROM THE SPECTACULAR RESTAURANT HE OWNS.

DaSilvano
ALEC BALDWIN LOVED THE SHOVEL-NOSE LOBSTER. I SAVED YOU ONE. COME OVER, I'M HUNGRY!

I USUALLY WAIT AT THE BAR FOR OUR TABLE AND WATCH THE ALL-SEEING, ALWAYS-MOVING SILVANO DO HIS THING.

NO CHEESE ON SEAFOOD PASTA! IT'S A SACRILEGE!

TAKE THE STUFF OUT OF YOUR APRON, YOU LOOK LIKE A KANGAROO!

'AVE THE OSSO BUCO. IT'S THE END OF THE WORLD!

THIS ALL HAPPENED IN THE SAME MINUTE, I SWEAR.

THE MOST ENERGETIC MAN ON THE PLANET FINALLY SITS DOWN, AND I TELL HIM ABOUT MY WONDERFUL DAY.

SILVANO, THE DOCTOR ASPIRATED A LUMP IN MY BREAST AND I GET THE RESULTS TOMORROW, BUT DON'T WORRY...

...THERE'S A CHANCE IT MAY *NOT* BE CANCEROUS.

THE NEXT DAY, FRIDAY, MAY 14, I WAS SUPPOSED TO GET THE RESULTS, SO WHENEVER I HEARD...

RING! RING!

WAAA-AHH!

WHOOSH!

THUD!

OUCH.

R E P E A T **57** T I M E S

IT'S YOUR MOMMA, ANYONE CALL?.
...ABOUT CANCER?

CONVERSATION #4, 5, 6, 9, 10, 11, 12, 13, 14, 16, 17, 18, 19, 20, 21, 23, 24, 25, 26, 27, 29, 35, 44, 45, 46, 47, 48, 51, 52, 55 & 56

MARISA, GIRL... ANY WORD...
...ABOUT CANCER?

SHARON WORE LATEX GLOVES AND A MASK WHILE COLORING HAIR

CONVERSATION #15, 43

ANYTING NEW...
...ABOUT CANCER?

CONVERSATION #1, 3, 8, 22, 38, 39, 41, 49, 57

MAY 14 PHONE LOG:

TOTAL # OF INCOMING CALLS: 57

TOTAL # OF CALLS FROM SILVANO: 9

TOTAL # OF CALLS FROM MY BFFs: 17

TOTAL # OF CALLS FROM MY (S)MOTHER: 31

TOTAL # OF CALLS FROM DOCTORS: 0

'EY BABY, 'OW DOES THIS LOOK?

IT CLASHES, SO I LOVE IT.

OK-FAR-OUT-I-LOVE-YOU-GOO'BYE.

I LOVE YOU TOO, GOO'BYE.

CALL-ME-IF-YOU-'EAR-ANYTING-OR-IF-YOU-NEED-ANYTING.

I WON'T. WHAT DOCTOR CALLS ON THE WEEKEND?

10:03 A.M.

RING! RING!

IT'S-ME-I-FORGOT-MY-SUNGLASSES-I-GOTTA-GO-TO-WORK-CIAO!

CIAO, BELLO.

SCH-ZOOOSH!

RING! RING!

palmOne

T·Mobile

Dr. Mills Calling

10:12 A.M. EXACTLY.

MARISA, THIS IS DR. MILLS. THERE IS AN ABNORMALITY.

MY WORLD CAME TO AN END.

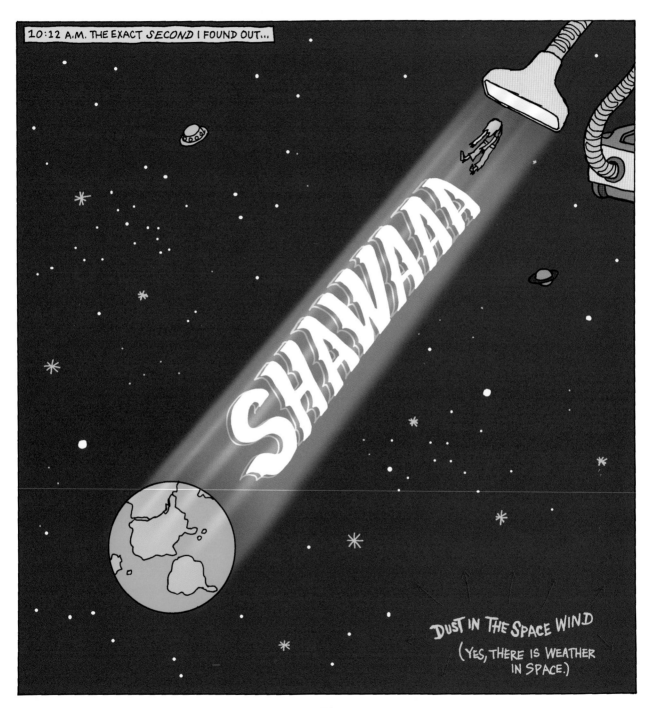

THE ELECTROLUX OF THE UNIVERSE SUCKED ME INTO A BLACK HOLE.

THUP!

I WAS ALONE.

AFRAID.

FROZEN IN TIME FOR AN ETERNITY IN A VAST EXPANSE OF NOTHINGNESS, SURROUNDED BY DARK MATTER...

...WISHING I COULD JUST GO BACK TO WORRYING ABOUT MY STUPID, SELF-ABSORBED, SELF-ESTEEM, WEIGHT, BAD-SKIN, BAD HAIR ISSUES THAT HAD OBSESSED ME MY WHOLE LIFE...

NOW, WHO KNEW IF I'D EVEN *HAVE* HAIR?

I AM NOWHERE

OR IF I'D EVEN LIVE?

10:12:03 A.M. THE NEXT MILLISECOND. I HAD TO CALL MY PARENTS...

OF COURSE MY (S)MOTHER PICKED UP THE PHONE FIRST.

OHMYGOD, I'M SICK!

THE JERSEY SHORE

IF MY DAD HATED THE PHONE BEFORE...

MOM JUST RAN INTO THE TUSH.

MARISA, DON'T TELL ME!

OH GOD OH GOD OH GOD OH GOD PLEASE GOD NO!

LA TOILETTE

WHY DO I HAVE CANCER NOW? WHY DO I NEED A LUMPECTOMY NOW? WHY IS THIS HAPPENING NOW? NOW WHEN I'VE NEVER BEEN HAPPIER!

YOU HAVE TO TELL SILVANO RIGHT NOW. HE'S GOING TO BE YOUR HUSBAND.

HON, GET ME THE EXTENSION!

I'M AFRAID TO TELL SILVANO...

MARISA, IT'S MOM. SILVANO IS A MAN OF GREAT CHARACTER.

THIS IS DAD, HON. HE'S NOT JUST ANY MAN, AND THAT'S WHY YOU WAITED 43 YEARS TO GET MARRIED.

BUT WHEN WOMEN GET SICK MEN LEAVE. HUSBANDS LEAVE THEIR WIVES... AND WE'RE NOT EVEN MARRIED!

BUT MAY 15, 2004, WASN'T THE FIRST TIME IN MY LIFE THAT THINGS WERE GREAT AND THEN SUDDENLY...

YOU KNOW, I WASN'T ALWAYS
THE SELF-AWARE NARCISSIST
I AM TODAY...

I'M NOT SAYING THE *FABULISTA* LIFE WASN'T FUN. IT WAS. MY BFF BOB AND I WENT TO ALL THE "IT" EVENTS.

FABULOUS. FABULOUS.

WHO WOULDN'T LOVE THE FRONT ROW OF A FASHION SHOW?

PEOPLE WHO AREN'T IN THEM.

...AND WE WENT TO ALL THE "IT" PARTIES.

THERE'S SARAH JESSICA...PHEW! FOR A MOMENT I THOUGHT THERE WAS *NOBODY* HERE!

AFTER 1 OR 10 DIRTY MARTINIS, FASHION COMMENTATOR BOB TURNED HIS ATTENTION TO YOURS TRULY...

LOOK AT YOU...TOO MUCH BLUE EYESHADOW AND TOO MUCH GLITTER IN THAT BLUE EYE SHADOW...

...LOUD SILVER PLATFORMS WITH *LOUDER* ORANGE PANTS...

...AND I WON'T EVEN COMMENT ON THE AQUA FROST TOENAIL COLOR.

ALL THIS FROM A MAN IN AN IRIDESCENT PURPLE PRADA SUIT!

IT'S A *BLUE* VIOLET. TO BE OF *FASHION* IS TO BE COLD. YOU TRY TOO HARD.

THIS IS THE NEXT THING BOB SAID:

I WOULD HAVE BEEN ANNOYED HAD I NOT GOTTEN A CARTOON OUT OF IT.

THAT'S BASED ON ME

THAT IS BOB

"Stop smiling. You're downtown."

ONE DAY THAT AUGUST, DREW LEE, MY EDITOR AT *TALK* MAGAZINE, ASKED ME TO DO A STORY ON HOW TO BE AN "IT" GIRL...

Talk MEDIA

THERE ARE EXPERTS THE "IT" GIRLS GO TO. I WANT A PIECE ABOUT *THEM*. AND I WANT TO GET THE NUMBERS... HOW MUCH DOES IT *REALLY* COST?

TALK MAGAZINE IS NO LONGER, MAY IT R.I.P.

MAYBE THOSE EXPERTS CAN GIVE ME A FEW TIPS.

DREW, I'M ON THE STREET, HANG ON WHILE I FIND A PEN.

THIS PEN DOESN'T WORK!

THIS PEN DOESN'T WORK!

THIS PEN DOESN'T WORK!

AN ARTIST THAT DOESN'T HAVE *ANY* WORKING PENS...

WHY DO THEY MAKE THE *INSIDES* OF HANDBAGS BLACK SO YOU CAN *NEVER* SEE ANYTHING?!?!

HANG ON HANG ON HANG ON...

OK, DREW.

I *FINALLY* FOUND A PEN THAT WRITES... SHOOT.

TALK TO THE "IT" PERSONAL TRAINER, THE "IT" DERMATOLOGIST SLASH MEDISPA, FIND THE "IT" BAG, THE "IT" WATCH...

DREW EATS GUMMI BEARS FOR LUNCH

...THEN ADD UP EVERYTHING YOU'D SPEND SO WE HAVE A GRAND TOTAL AT THE END AND WE'LL KNOW "WHAT 'IT' COSTS."

HE PREFERS CHERRY

BY THE WAY MARISA, TINA LOVES THIS STORY... GO FOR IT!

CLICK!

THAT'S TINA BROWN, THE EDITOR IN CHIEF.

1 DEFORESTED RAIN FOREST LATER, I RANG MY *THEN* BOYFRIEND, THE ACTOR...

HEY, GUESS WHO GOT A BRAZILIAN BIKINI WAX...

I COULD COME...

...OVER.

BEEP!

I WASN'T SURPRISED HE DIDN'T PICK UP. HE WAS SO SELF-ABSORBED, HE *NEVER* PICKED UP ON ANYTHING.

5TH AVE

THANK GOD FOR CALL WAITING...

I JUST GOT A CANCELLATION, MAREESE, HOW GOES IT?

THE MADISON AVENUE SALON WHERE "IT" HAIRCOLORIST SHARON WORKS.

THE PURSUIT OF "IT" IS DRIVING ME NUTS! I HAVEN'T FOUND THE "IT" BAG, THE "IT" WATCH, THE "IT" PHONE-- BUT I DO HAVE THE "IT" COLLAGEN, LIPOSUCTION, FAT INJECTIONS, LIP AUGMENTATIONS, EXFOLIATIONS, DERMABRASIONS, BOTOX, ELECTROSHOCK CELLULITE REMOVAL, ELECTROSHOCK FACIALS, STRING FACIALS, LASER FACIALS, FOOT FACIALS, LASER FOOT FACIALS, LASER COLLAGEN SOFT PILLOWS IN THE BALLS OF YOUR FEET, MEDIPEELS, MEDIPEDIS, MEDIMANIS, EYEBROWS TINTED, INDIVIDUAL FALSE EYELASHES APPLIED 1 AT A TIME, EYELASH TINTING, EYELASH PERMING, LASER HAIR REMOVAL, TIT JOB, NOSE JOB, BUT YOU NEED IT BECAUSE IN THIS TOWN YOU'RE EITHER A NOBODY OR A GREAT BODY AND IT ALREADY COSTS $179,546 AND I'M NOT EVEN DONE WITH IT. YOU GET 1 THING DONE THEN ANOTHER THING DONE. THIS IS AN ENDLESS SLIPPERY SLOPE CHASING THE UNATTAINABLE "IT" AND AS SOON AS YOU HAVE "IT"-- IT'S GONE! IT'S CRAZY!

THAT'S HOW GOES IT!

SHARON'S STATION, 11 MINUTES LATER:

DOING THE *BEAUTY* STORY HAS MADE ME FEEL REALLY *UGLY*... THE EXPERTS FOUND FLAWS I DIDN'T EVEN KNOW I HAD!

YOU'RE LOOKING A LITTLE MOUSEY.

COST: $450 FOR HIGHLIGHTS

OH SHARON... NOT YOU, TOO!

I GUESS IT'S THE NATURE OF THE BEAUTY BEAST!

WHY ARE YOU COMPLAINING? IF YOU WRITE ABOUT IT, YOU GET TO HAVE IT, THAT'S HOW THE BUSINESS WORKS...AS LONG AS YOUR PIECE IS PRINTED.

SCRATCH MY BACK, I'LL WAX, NIP, TUCK, PLUCK, BLEACH YOURS?

RING! RING!

GOOD LUCK FINDING ANYTHING IN THIS BAG.

OH, HERE IT IS...

IT'S MY NEXT APPOINTMENT.

Da Silvano Connected

SO OFF I WENT TO INTERVIEW THE "IT" RESTAURATEUR, SILVANO MARCHETTO. IT JUST SO HAPPENS THAT THE "IT" RESTAURANT HAS BEEN MY "IT" PLACE SINCE I WAS 17.

Da Sil

SILVANO, HOW DO I GET AN "A"* TABLE?

*FYI: YOU WOULD NEVER SAY "IT" TABLE, YOU JUST WOULDN'T.

MARISA, EVERY TABLE'S AN "A" TABLE.

KITCHEN

BAR

ANTIPASTO TABLE

WINES

DA SILVANO FLOOR PLAN

C'MON. THIS IS AN "A" TABLE?

MADONNA WAS 'ERE LAST NIGHT AND SHE SAT IN YOUR SEAT.

MADONNA SAT HERE? WHO WAS SHE WITH? WHAT DID SHE EAT?

GUY RITCHIE AND SHE 'AD THE LAMB CHOP AND SAID IT WAS FANTASTIC.

MAYBE SOME OF HER MADONNA-NESS WILL RUB OFF ON ME.

20

JUST AS KIMBERLEY AND MARION WERE GETTING IN MY FACE ABOUT MY "BEAUTIFUL, UNIQUE" NOSE...

OK, I'M GOING TO BRING OUT A FEW DISHES...

CAVAILLON MELONS FLOWN IN FROM FRANCE WITH PORT WINE.

GREEN 'EIRLOOM TOMATOES, THEY'RE BETTER THAN RED.

OUVOLI MUSHROOM SALAD. THEY'RE IN SEASON; DON'T THEY LOOK LIKE EGGS?

DIVINE.

FANTASTIC.

WHAT A FEAST.

I'M NOT JOKING, I THOUGHT THERE WERE 4 SILVANOS...

AND WE DRANK...

...SPECTACULAR SUPER TUSCAN RED WINE...

WE HAD DOVER SOLE, GNOCCHI WITH LOBSTER SAUCE,* PANNA COTTA** WITH CHOCOLATE SAUCE AND LIMONCELLO***

AND WE DRANK...

IT WAS POSITIVELY ORGASMIC!

* GNOCCHI ARE POTATO DUMPLINGS ** PANNA COTTA IS BAKED CREAM *** LIMONCELLO IS LEMON LIQUER FROM CAPRI

WOULD YOU LIKE ANYTING ELSE?

ARE YOU KIDDING? THIS WAS THE MOST I'VE EATEN ALL YEAR. WE'LL JUST TAKE THE CHECK.

THERE IS NO CHECK.

THERE IS NO CHECK?

NO!

JUST-TAKE-CARE-OF-MY-GUYS-TANK-YOU!

OF COURSE WE WILL, THANK YOU.

BUT YOU'RE THE ONE WHO TOOK CARE OF US.

UHHUH. WHY DID HE COMP DINNER?

I HAVEN'T BEEN COMPED IN SO LONG I FORGOT WHAT IT FEELS LIKE.

MARISA WAKE UP, THAT ACTOR'S NEVER GOING TO MARRY YOU! DON'T GIVE UP ON YOUR DREAM TO HAVE KIDS!

Garden State Parkway ↓

MOM, I'LL HAVE KIDS WHEN I'M READY! WHAT TIME IS IT? I CAN'T BE LATE!

YOU'RE ALREADY LATE... FOR MOTHERHOOD!

TELL SHARON TO MAKE YOU A LITTLE LIGHTER... THE VIRGIN MARY THINKS YOU'RE STILL TOO DARK!

THE VIRGIN MARY IS A BEAUTY EXPERT TOO?! BEFORE SHE WAS A CARTOONIST, AND THE NEW YORKER WASN'T BUYING HER EITHER...

MA, I GOTTA GO!

THAT'S NOT FUNNY, MISSY! I'M BUSY TOO, YOU KNOW...

YOUR SISTER'S TRYING TO CON ME INTO BABYSITTING JOHNNY, BUT GRANDMA'S NOT WATCHING HIM UNTIL HE DOES POOPY IN THE POTTY!

EYE, YI, YI! BYE, I LOVE YOU, MA.

BYE, I LOVE YOU, HON.

HANDICAPPED PARKING

SLAM!

NO ONE EVER LISTENS TO ME.

THE OFFICES OF *THE NEW YORKER* ARE AT 4 TIMES SQUARE. I ARRIVED AT 11:38 A.M.

HOME OF *VOGUE, GQ, VANITY FAIR, GLAMOUR,* THE CONDÉ NAST BUILDING IS THE CENTER OF THE MEDIA UNIVERSE.

THE LOBBY IS POPULATED BY "IT" GIRLS, MOST OF THEM ARE *MAGAZISTAS.*

I FELT LIKE AN ALIEN AND I LIKED IT.

I JUMPED INTO THE ELEVATOR AND BUMPED INTO JENNIFER...

HI. HI.

RIVAL CARTOON GIRL

SHE AND I HAD BEEN RIVALS IN ADVERTISING FOR YEARS...

IS SHE NOW SUBMITTING TO *THE NEW YORKER?!*

20

NEXT I GOT IN LINE FOR MY INDIVIDUAL MEETING WITH BOB MANKOFF, THE CARTOON EDITOR. IT'S FIRST COME, FIRST SEEN.

SAM, AKA "S. GROSS" IS MY BFF

EVERY WEEK SOMEONE WHO COMES IN AFTER ME TRIES TO CUT THE LINE.

I'M SORRY I'M SORRY I'M SORRY I'M LATE.

NOW THAT YOU'RE HERE, LET'S GO TO O'LUNNEY'S.

WE ATE AT O'LUNNEY'S LAST WEEK.

I WANT TO GO TO PERGOLA, LET'S WALK OVER NOW.

I'LL WAIT FOR YOU, KIDDO.

DON'T EVEN *THINK* ABOUT IT, MORT.

I WOULDN'T DREAM OF IT, MARISA.

TAP! TAP!

FINALLY IT WAS MY TURN TO FACE REJECTION...

HI BOB, HOW 'BOUT THOSE YANKS?

BOB MANKOFF BROUGHT ME UP INTO THE MAJORS, AND FOR THAT I'M ETERNALLY GRATEFUL.

BOB HOLDS 3 CARTOONS OUT OF MY BATCH OF 12. I HAVEN'T HAD AN "OK" IN WEEKS AND MY BATTING AVERAGE IS SINKING.

YOUR WOMEN ARE TOO THIN, TOO PRETTY, THEY'RE NOT REAL AND I CAN'T RELATE TO THEM.

MY REJECTS

GO TO THE LOBBY OF THIS BUILDING, TAKE A WALK OUTSIDE, EAT AT A RESTAURANT DOWNTOWN... LOOK BOB, OPEN YOUR EYES, THIS IS *THE NEW YORKER,* I'M DRAWING *REAL* NEW YORKERS.

I'M A WUSS.

I REALLY DIDN'T SAY THAT.

DON'T WORRY ABOUT *THE NEW YORKER*. LISTEN, LAST WEEK I WAS DOING *CAT GAGS*, NOW I'M ONTO CHICKENS. IF HE DOESN'T BUY THEM, I'LL HIT THE STREETS AND FIND SOMEONE WHO WILL. DO YOU KNOW WHY?

WHY?

BECAUSE I'M A STREET RAT.

STREET RATS KNOW HOW TO SURVIVE ON THE STREETS, OUTSIDE IN THE ELEMENTS.

MAYBE YOU SHOULD TRY DRAWING DOGS.

DOGS?!

CARTOONISTS LOVED PERGOLA. IT WASN'T FANCY AND THE PRICE WAS RIGHT.

PLUS THEY GAVE US A FREE GLASS OF WINE

ROOKIE, AT LEAST *YOU'RE* NOT BEING PHASED OUT.

WHAT ARE YOU TALKING ABOUT? YOU GUYS ARE THE MASTERS!

THEY'RE NOT BUYING FROM US ANYMORE.

I DON'T KNOW FROM THESE NEW CARTOON-ISTS.

MAY I SAY SOMETHING?

IF YOU *MUST.*

C'MON, GIVE SOMEONE ELSE THE FLOOR.

WELL, I HAVE THIS COUSIN WHO CALLS ME TO FIND OUT WHO IN MY FAMILY IS STILL ALIVE...

...I HADN'T BEEN PRINTED IN *THE NEW YORKER* IN A WHILE...

...SO THIS WEEK SHE PHONED ME...

...TO FIND OUT WHETHER I WAS DEAD.

THEN, ANOTHER MONDAY NIGHT A FEW WEEKS LATER.
SEPTEMBER 11, 3:06 A.M.
I WAS ON DEADLINE FOR *THE NEW YORKER*, WATCHING MY PARENTS' YORKIE WHILE THEY WERE AWAY.

8:47 A.M. I WAS WOKEN OUT OF A DEEP SLEEP.

MAN, THAT WAS ONE LOUD PLANE...

THE JET SOUNDED LIKE IT FLEW RIGHT OVER MY APARTMENT.

12 MINUTES LATER...

IT'S KIMBERLEY— NEW YORK IS UNDER ATTACK! COME TO CONNECTICUT RIGHT NOW!

I CAN'T, I HAVE PRECIOUS AND I HAVE TO GO TO THE NEW YORKER!

THERE IS NO NEW YORKER!

KIMBERLEY WAS RIGHT. *THE NEW YORKER* WAS SHUT DOWN. IMMEDIATELY AFTER THE FIRST PLANE HIT, I SAW PEOPLE COVERED WITH DUST RUNNING UP THE STREETS FROM DOWNTOWN.

COUGH! COUGH!

COUGH!

I RUSHED HOME, WORRIED ABOUT PRECIOUS'S LITTLE LUNGS.

1:32 P.M. MY *TALK* EDITOR DREW CALLED ME ON MY LAND LINE. CELL PHONES DIDN'T WORK BECAUSE THE ANTENNA WAS ON TOP OF TOWER 2.

MARISA, WE'RE RIPPING APART THE MAGAZINE AND WE'RE SENDING EVERYONE TO GROUND ZERO... CAN YOU COVER IT FROM YOUR END?!?!

...AND BY THE WAY, YOUR STORY "WHAT 'IT' COSTS" IS DEAD. IT'S TOO SUPERFICIAL RIGHT NOW.

EVERYTHING IS SUPERFICIAL RIGHT NOW.

OK PRECIOUS, I'LL SEE YOU IN A BIT.

SOB! SOB!

SOB! SOB!

THEN I GRABBED MY TAPE RECORDER, CAMERA, FILM, BLANK TAPES, PENS AND SKETCH PAD AND TREKKED DOWNTOWN TO GROUND ZERO...

I REMEMBER SEEING EVERYONE WAS IN A DAZE.

ON HUDSON STREET, HUNDREDS OF PEOPLE TOOK PICTURES OF GROUND ZERO 6 BLOCKS AWAY.

AT FIRST I THOUGHT IT WAS ODD, BUT NOW I THINK IT'S IMPORTANT WE *NEVER* FORGET.

THE NATIONAL GUARD KNEW EARLY ON...

THEY SENT US DOWN TO "SEARCH AND RESCUE," BUT IT'S REALLY "SEARCH AND RECOVER!"

I DIDN'T UNDERSTAND THEIR LINGO, BUT NOW WE ALL KNOW WHAT THAT MEANS.

6:30. I WENT HOME TO FEED PRECIOUS.

I KNOW, HONEY, I'M TOO UPSET TO EAT, TOO.

10:00 P.M. I FINALLY WENT HOME.

I DIDN'T WEAR A MASK, ALTHOUGH THE ACRID SMELL AND THE AMOUNT OF PARTICLES IN THE AIR WAS STAGGERING.

SEPTEMBER 12. I RAN THE ART OVER TO *TALK* MAGAZINE, AND SAW THE DESIGNER TOM FORD AND HIS BOYFRIEND IN CRISP WHITE SHIRTS AND NOT A WRINKLE IN THEIR PRESSED JEANS

THERE WERE NO CARS ON 6TH AVENUE AND THE SUBWAYS WEREN'T WORKING.

13TH ST   6TH

I GUESS EVERYONE HAD THEIR OWN WAY OF KEEPING IT TOGETHER...

...MY WAY WAS TO KEEP WORKING.

I MADE IT TO *TALK* MINUTES BEFORE THEY WENT TO PRESS.

HERE YOU GO, DREW.

THE WHOLE MAGAZINE WAS IN TEARS.

HERE'S WHAT RAN IN *TALK* MAGAZINE.
(IT'S STILL ONE OF
THE THINGS I'M MOST PROUD OF.)

WEEKS AFTER, THE ACRID SMELL CONTINUED TO BLANKET DOWNTOWN...

MAYBE YOU SHOULD LEAVE THE CITY FOR A WHILE, I'VE SEEN MORE CASES OF *ASTHMA* SINCE 9/11.

I HAVE *ASTHMA*?!
≋COUGH!≋
≋COUGH!≋
≋COUGH!≋

LUNG SPECIALIST DR. PAT TIETJIN

THERE WAS ASBESTOS, BENZENE AND GOD KNOWS WHAT ELSE WAS IN THE AIR BACK THEN... AND EVEN *SHE* DOESN'T WANT TO THINK ABOUT IT.

SO WHEN I FIRST GOT THE DIAGNOSIS... **FAST FORWARD**

WE'RE JUMPING AHEAD TO **2004**...

I ASKED THE NUMBER 1 QUESTION:

IS *THAT* WHY I GOT CANCER?!

9/11 COULD BE A FACTOR, BUT MARISA...

...DO YOU REALLY WANT TO DRIVE YOURSELF CRAZY PLAYING *THAT* GAME?!

YOU THINK THIS IS A *GAME*?!

RESEARCH HEAD
"STUDIES SUGGEST THAT IT DOES INCREASE THIS RISK."

MOVE RIGHT **4** SPACES

"I EAT A LOT OF TAKEOUT, WHAT ABOUT THE COATING IN THE CONTAINERS?"

MOVE BACK **3** SPACES

RESEARCH HEAD "YES, THERE IS DATA THAT CONFIRMS THIS DOES INCREASE THE RISK."

MOVE UP **4** SPACES

I GOT MY PERIOD WHEN I WAS 11

WHAT IF YOU HAD A LATE MENOPAUSE?

MOVE BACK **1** SPACE

RESEARCH HEAD

MOVE BAC

WHEN I WAS 40, I HAD MY FIRST CHILD.

I NEVER HAD CHILDREN.

MOVE BACK **3** SPACES

THAT CHEMICAL IS ALSO ON TEFLON PANS

THE CA GUESSIN
'ROUND AND 'ROUND AND 'ROUND

RESEARCH HEAD
"IT IS LIKELY TO CAUSE BREAST CANCER."

MOVE UP **12** SPACES

"DOES HAVING A DRINK OR 3 EVERY NIGHT PUT ME AT RISK?"

MOVE BACK **5** SPACES

"MY MOTHER HAD BREAST CANCER, DO I HAVE THE GENE?"

MOVE BACK **6** SPACES

"DO PESTICIDES HAVE ANYTHING TO DO WITH BREAST CANCER?"

MOVE BACK **5** SPACES

"WOMEN WHO STOPPED USING THE PILL MORE THAN 10 YEARS AGO DO NOT SEEM TO HAVE AN INCREASED RISK, BUT IF YOU TOOK THE HIGHER DOSES IN THE LATE 70s, YOU COULD STILL BE AT RISK."

RESEARCH HEAD

MOVE UP **9** SPACES

"I SMOKED AND NOW I HAVE BREAST CANCER... COINCIDENCE?"

MOVE BACK **7** SPACES

CORPORATE HEAD

MOVE UP

AS I LOOKED AT ALL THE SUPPOSED FACTORS THAT CONTRIBUTED TO ANY BREAST CANCER DIAGNOSIS...
THE PILL, HORMONES IN BEEF, DAIRY AND POULTRY, RADIATION, OVEREATING, THIS LIST COULD GO ON INTO INFINITY...
IT STRUCK ME THAT 99% OF THE REASONS ARE CREATED BY HUMAN BEINGS...

WHAT THE HELL ARE WE *DOING* TO OURSELVES?!

MARISA, REMEMBER US...

...WE'RE FROM THE BREAST CANCER AND LEUKEMIA CLUSTER 20 MILES FROM YOUR PARENTS' SHORE HOUSE.

WE THINK IT WAS CAUSED BY THE POWER LINES NEAR OUR SCHOOL. WE WERE ALL CLASSMATES...

...BUT OUR RITZY TOWN KEPT IT QUIET. THEY DIDN'T WANT THEIR REAL E$TATE PRICE$ TO DROP.

WAIT... DON'T FORGET US!

36

A MOMENT OF SILENCE.

WHEN YOU LIGHT A CANDLE,
YOU ILLUMINATE A SOUL.

ABOUT THAT LOUSY RELATIONSHIP? I ADMIT VALENTINE'S DAY IS A DUMB COMMERCIAL HOLIDAY, BUT...

MY GIFT TO YOU IS THESE CHOCOLATES.

I BOUGHT THE ACTOR A ONE POUND BOX FROM VARGANO'S, WEST VILLAGE'S FINEST

MY GIFT TO YOU IS THIS MEAL.

THE MEAL WAS A PIZZA, WE WERE AT A PIZZERIA AND HE TOOK THE BIGGER HALF...

I GUESS I COULD'VE ACCEPTED THAT, WE SPLIT EVERY MEAL WHEN....

RING! RING!

THE CELL PHONE I BOUGHT HIM,

MA! DID YOU GET THE FLOWERS I SENT YOU?

BOY OH BOY DID I GET A WAKE-UP CALL OR WHAT???!!!

FLOWERS?!

HE WAS PUTTIN' OUT FOR HIS MOTHER!

BLUE SKIES SMILIN' AT ME...

SING IT WITH ME, MA!

HERE'S SOMETHING ABOUT ACTORS...THEY'RE ALWAYS SINGING...IN PUBLIC!

SO, HE THOUGHT HE WAS MY LEADING MAN...

TAXI!

IRONICALLY, THE BREAKUP HAPPENED IN THE JEWELRY DISTRICT.

...BUT HE WAS JUST A 2-MINUTE WALK-ON IN THE MOVIE OF MY LIFE.

DRIVER, CARMINE STREET AND STEP ON IT!

THAT NIGHT, I GOT HOME AND...

SLAM!

...SHUT THAT DOOR SO HARD PLEASE GOD MARY JESUS JOSEPH YAHWEH BUDDHA ALLAH ATHENA DON'T EVER LET IT OPEN AGAIN!

FEBRUARY 15, I HAD A MEETING WITH SILVANO...

I'D DRAWN UP 4 IDEAS, HOPEFULLY HE'D LIKE 1...

LET'S DO THEM,

WHICH 1 OF THEM?

ALL OF THEM.

THERE'S 4 OF THEM.

I KNOW, I WANT ALL 4 OF THEM.

FOR THE RECORD, I NEVER STOPPED WEARING THIS EYE SHADOW...

1 WEEK LATER, I BROUGHT THE FINAL ART.

WE CHANGED THE NAME OF THE RESTAURANT. CAN YOU CHANGE IT?

SURE, I'LL DO IT.

1 WEEK LATER, I BROUGHT THE FINAL ART.

WE CHANGED THE LIGHTS IN THE RESTAURANT. CAN YOU CHANGE IT?

SURE, I'LL CHANGE THEM.

...ALL 4 OF THEM.

1 WEEK LATER, I BROUGHT THE FINAL ART.

PERFECT-PERFECT-PERFECT-TANK YOU VERY MUCH.

YOU'RE WELCOME, INVITE ME TO THE OPENING.

SEE YA 'ROUND, SILVANO. IT WAS A PLEASURE DOING BUSINESS WITH YOU.

TANK YOU, TANK YOU.

FINISHING UP THE CARDS WAS BITTERSWEET...

WHO'S GOING TO DATE YOU NOW, MISS ORANGE PANTS?

BOB, I KINDA HAVE A CRUSH ON SILVANO... AND HE WEARS ORANGE PANTS.

FASHION TIP #1: DON'T TAKE EVERY FASHION TIP.

OK, WELL.

I REALLY HATE IT WHEN GAY COUPLES DRESS LIKE TWINS.

YOU BETTER NOT DATE SILVANO! IF THINGS DON'T WORK OUT, AND CONSIDERING YOUR TERRIBLE TRACK RECORD THEY WON'T... WE WON'T BE ABLE TO GET A TABLE THERE!

WE LOVE DASILVANO AND WE DON'T WANT YOU TO RUIN IT FOR US!

LISA IS THE BEAUTY-PRODUCTS QUEEN

DID I TELL YOU THAT SHARON AND LISA WERE MY BFFs?

BUT I WASN'T OFF THE HOOK JUST YET...AND I KINDA LIKED IT.

MARISA, SILVANO... CAN YOU CHANGE THE DATE OF THE OPENING?

MARISA, SILVANO.... CAN YOU CHANGE THE HOURS?

MARISA, SILVANO... CAN YOU FIND A PRINTER?

ON THE FIRST WARM DAY IN MARCH, I FOUND SILVANO BASKING IN THE SUN OUTSIDE...

AHH...CHE BELLA GIORNATA!

HE WAS WORKING ON HIS TAN

SILVANO, THE CARDS ARE READY.

VINO ROSSO PER MARISA!

DO YOU LIKE THEM?

I *LOVE* THEM.

SO MARISA, I JUST GOT A NEW MASERATI.

CONGRATULATIONS, YOU DESERVE IT.

HERE'S YOUR RED WINE.

IT'S YELLOW, AND I'M GETTING ANOTHER MASERATI IN BLUE.

I'M SO HAPPY FOR YOU. I SEE HOW HARD YOU WORK.

MARISA, I SEE 'OW 'ARD *YOU* WORK, AND...

...I'D LIKE TO OFFER YOU MY 'OUSE IN FLORIDA FOR A WEEK.

THAT'S VERY GENEROUS, BUT NO THANKS, SILVANO.

THEN LET ME OFFER YOU MY 'OUSE IN TUSCANY FOR A WEEK...

I LOVE FLORENCE, BUT ACTUALLY, HERE'S WHAT I WOULD REALLY LIKE...

MY PARENTS BROUGHT ME HERE WHEN I WAS 17. I'D LIKE TO GIFT THEM WITH A MEAL.

I DON'T KNOW IF I EVER TOLD YOU THIS...

MY GREAT-GRANDFATHER AND HIS BROTHER WERE CHEFS... ...AND HE STARTED ONE OF THE FIRST ITALIAN RESTAURANTS HERE IN 1901.

IT WAS CALLED "NICOLA'S." THAT'S HIM IN THE CHEF'S HAT ↓

REALLY? I DIDN'T KNOW THAT!

OK, THEN. IN THE NEXT FEW WEEKS I'LL BRING MY PARENTS FOR LUNCH.

DEAL?

DEAL.

DOING THE DA SILVANO CARDS WAS FUN, BUT I REALLY NEEDED A PAYING JOB...

LIKE STREET RAT SAM SAYS, CARTOONISTS HAVE TO POUND THE PAVEMENT TO FIND SCRAPS OF WORK.

GLAMOUR

GLAMOUR GIRLS WILL START RUNNING IN MAY.

I GOT A MONTLY CARTOON IN THE *DOS, DON'TS* SECTION. WOO HOO!

LATER THAT WEEK, SAM AND I WENT TO A *NEW YORKER* PARTY.

YA DID GOOD, KIDDO.

I'M ALSO WORKING ON A TV PILOT. IF IT DOESN'T GO I'LL LOSE MY WRITERS GUILD INSURANCE.

C'MON SAM... LET'S GET INTO PARTY MODE.

SNAP!

LET'S GET MORE BOOZE.

MUSIC TO MY EARS.

HEY MARISA....

WANNA DANCE?

OH, GO AHEAD.

MITCH WAS JUST A CARTOON COMRADE, I DIDN'T THINK ANYTHING OF IT UNTIL...

HEY MARISA...

IT WAS JENNIFER, RIVAL CARTOON GIRL...

45

YOU'RE A STUPID ★★★★ING ★★★★ !!!*

*SORRY, I DON'T WANT THOSE UGLY WORDS OF RIVAL CARTOON GIRL IN MY BOOK.

I HATE YOU BECAUSE YOU ALWAYS HAVE A BOYFRIEND!

WHAT THE HELL DID I START?

...AND BECAUSE YOU CAN WEAR LEATHER PANTS!

WHAT GRADE ARE YOU IN?!?

C'MON, LET'S GO.

WHAT GRADE WAS I IN?

COME ON, I'M SEPARATING YOU TWO...

WHAT THE HELL IS YOUR PROBLEM?

BUT I WILL SAY THAT I'VE NEVER BEEN CALLED ANYTHING LIKE THAT, EVER.

BACK THEN, ON A SCALE OF 1 TO 10 OF THE TERRIBLE THINGS THAT HAPPEN IN LIFE, THIS WAS AN 11. I HATED THAT WE WERE SO UNPROFESSIONAL AT A NEW YORKER PARTY, THE MAGAZINE WE BOTH KILLED OURSELVES TO GET INTO. I HATED HAVING A NEMESIS, AND I HATED HOW WOMEN HATE EACH OTHER IN BUSINESS.

THERE ARE OVER 50 MALE CARTOONISTS, AND I DON'T SEE YOU GUYS GETTING INTO CAT FIGHTS.

DIFFEE, I'M GONNA SCRATCH YOUR EYES OUT.

SHUT UP, ERIC.

SPEAKING OF CREATING A SCENE, SILVANO PUT UP HIS NEW SHINGLE, AND MY FRIENDS AND I HAD AN 8 O'CLOCK RESERVATION...

IT WAS AN AUTOMATIC HOT SPOT. THERE WAS A WAIT...

WHEN I GOT THERE, SILVANO TOOK ME AROUND...

MARISA, THIS IS MY DAUGHTER LEYLA, AND MY LAWYER, STEVE GARDNER. I WANTED THEM TO MEET YOU.

HELLO. HELLO. HELLO.

THEN MY FRIEND ANN ARRIVED, AND WE WERE SEATED.

LISA AND GRACIE ARE RUNNING LATE. THEY'RE PROBABLY BLOW-DRYING THEIR HAIR AND YOU KNOW HOW LONG *THAT* TAKES.

YEARS, AND SILVANO HATES IT WHEN YOU HOLD A TABLE.

LISA, HURRY UP, SILVANO DOES ANOTHER SEATING AT 10:00 AND IT'S 9:38!

FINALLY, AT 10:32:

HEY BABE!

TRAFFIC WAS AWFUL!

BALONEY!

WE'RE BLAMING IT ON THE BLOW-DRY.

THIS IS FROM SILVANO, TRUFFLES IN ICE CREAM.

SOUNDS DELICIOUS,

IT'S THE 5TH PLATE HE SENT OUT.

HOW MUCH CAN WE EAT?

12:02. SILVANO, WHO *NEVER* SITS WITH ANYONE, SAT WITH US. I WAS SHOCKED.

CONGRATULATIONS, THIS PLACE IS *PACKED* AND THE FOOD IS —

MEET-ME-IN-FRONT-OF-THE-DELI-AT-12:30.

HA HA HA HA HA HA HA

12:30 A.M.

QUICK STOP DELI

HE WAS IN FRONT OF THE DELI LIKE HE SAID HE WOULD BE.

WE WENT UP TO HIS APARTMENT.

YOU KNOW, I THOUGHT YOU WERE GAY.

WHY, BECAUSE I DIDN'T THROW MYSELF AT YOU?

NO, BECAUSE YOU ALWAYS SHOWED UP WITH WOMEN.

AND I WAS SO HAPPY.

THE NEXT MORNING, I WAS SO FREAKED OUT.

I SLIPPED PAST A SLEEPING SILVANO AND PUT ON MY SLIDES.

CHANEL FROM 1994

HE CAME OUT INTO THE LIVING ROOM, ALL SILVER-FOXY AND LONG EYELASHES.

YOU'RE LEAVING? AREN'T YOU GOING TO COMB YOUR HAIR?

ARE YOU KIDDING? PEOPLE BUY PRODUCTS TO GET THIS LOOK.

BACK AT CARMINE STREET, THE PHONE WOKE ME OUT OF A DEEP SLEEP.

IT'S SILVANO I 'AD A LOVELY TIME, WOULD YOU LIKE TO 'AVE DINNER WITH ME TONIGHT?

I CAN'T TONIGHT I'M GOING TO NEW JERSEY FOR MY BROTHER'S BIRTHDAY MAYBE I CAN TOMORROW IT DEPENDS WHEN I GET BACK.

THAT WAS A TOTAL LIE, I NEEDED TO DIGEST THIS.

5 MINUTES LATER...

MARISA BABE IT'S KIMBERLEY, PICK UP!

THIS WASN'T A ONE-NIGHT STAND, YOU'VE KNOWN HIM LONGER THAN ANYBODY... CALL HIM BACK RIGHT NOW!

A MILLISECOND LATER:

WE COULD GO TO DA SILVANO, OR WE COULD GO SOMEWHERE ELSE..

HE WAS SUNBATHING ON HIS TERRACE, SUNTAN LOTION: EXTRA VIRGIN OLIVE OIL SPF: 0

I'D LIKE TO GET TO KNOW YOU OUTSIDE OF YOUR RESTAURANT,

OUR FIRST DATE WAS AT BLUE RIBBON BAKERY, WHERE WE WENT THE NEXT NIGHT.

SILVANO, YOU LOOK ADORABLE. I'VE NEVER SEEN YOU IN A SUIT.

I WAS ALL CASUAL IN JEANS. WAS THIS MORE SERIOUS THAN I THOUGHT?

WE WERE THE ONLY DINERS DOWNSTAIRS. THAT'S WHERE HE POPPED THE QUESTION:

DO YOU WANT TO GO STEADY WITH ME?

STEADY? THAT'S SO OLD-FASHIONED.

AND THAT'S WHAT WON ME OVER.

I'D LOVE TO GO STEADY WITH YOU.

DEAL?

DEAL.

OK, NOW WHAT SHOULD WE EAT?

49

DaSilvano

IF NEW YORK CITY IS HIGH SCHOOL, THIS IS ITS CAFETERIA*...

THE POPULAR GIRLS —THE "IT" GIRLS; THE DRAMA DEPARTMENT—"A" LIST ACTORS; THE MUSIC DEPARTMENT—ROCK STARS; THE JOCKS—HALL OF FAME ATHLETES; THE NEWSPAPER—THE MEDIA ELITE, GOSSIP MEISTERS AND BLOGGER MONGERS WHO WATCH AND OVERHEAR EVERYONE'S EVERY MOVE AND REPORT IT; THE A.V. SQUAD—FILM, TV AND RECORD EXECUTIVES; THE HOMECOMING KING? SILVANO. AND ME? AS "THE GIRLFRIEND" I WAS THE NEW KID IN TOWN. YOU KNOW WHAT THAT MEANS. THAT WAS MY BIGGEST CHALLENGE. HERE'S WHAT HAPPENED WHEN I WENT TO SCHOOL ...

✳ WITH FABULOUS FOOD, OF COURSE.

THE FASHION EDITOR HEADED FOR SILVANO WHO WAS AT A TABLE BY HIMSELF...

...BUT AS SOON AS I JOINED HIM...

...SHE WENT FOR MATT DILLON INSTEAD.

"THE MOZZARELLA FONDLER" DIPPED HER HAND IN CHEESY WATER WHILE HITTING ON SILVANO.

TOO BAD SHE MISSED THE 3 FOOT ZUCCHINI BEHIND HER. GROPING THAT WOULD HAVE BEEN EVEN SUBTLER.

THE PHOTOGRAPHER WANTED ME OUT OF THE PICTURE.

SILVANO, SILVANO...LET'S YOU AND ME GO TO BUNGALOW 8.

AM I FREAKING INVISIBLE?!

THE STOCK GIRL WANTED TO HANDLE SILVANO'S MONEY, TOO.

BUT IF I DOUBTED MY PLACE IN HIS LIFE, SILVANO WAS 100% CERTAIN.

THIS IS THE NICEST THING ANYONE EVER DID FOR ME.

AND WHY DO YOU TINK I DID IT?

MARISA

SILVANO

RISERVATO

THAT'S "RESERVED" IN ITALIAN

IN FACT, TWO MONTHS AFTER WE BEGAN DATING, I MOVED INTO HIS PLACE.

GIRLS, YOU'RE OUTNUMBERED.

HE'S THE ONLY STRAIGHT MAN ON THE PLANET WHO HAS MORE SHOES THAN I DO!

THAT WEEK, AS I MADE MY WAY TO THE RESTAURANT...

FAT

POSEUR

OH HOLY SPIRIT PLEASE PUT A BUBBLE OF WHITE LIGHT AROUND SILVANO AND ME...

LOSER

THEN WAITED FOR SILVANO...

THE BOTOXED BUTTLESS BLONDE BRIGADE

SIT DOWN WITH US.

NO THANK YOU.

ACKNOWLEDGE IS POWER.

MANTRA #2

GET OVER HERE, I WANT TO ASK YOU SOMETHING!

OK, BUT I'M NOT SITTING.

ENGAGE AND YOU WON'T BE ENGAGED.

MANTRA #3

I'M A MODEL, HOW DID YOU GET HIM?!

DO YOU WANT SOMETING ELSE?

THIS GIRL TOOK THE PRIZE...

...ALMOST.

WHAT WOMAN WOULDN'T HAVE A MELTDOWN OVER THAT?!?!

HOW CAN YOU DO THAT TO ANOTHER WOMAN?!

ALL MY FRIENDS ARE *MODELS* AND WE'VE BEEN HITTING ON SILVANO FOR *15 YEARS!* HOW DID *YOU* GET HIM?

HOW DID *I* GET HIM?

RRRIP!

BY BEING A *GOOD* PERSON.

THWOP!

OF COURSE I REALLY DIDN'T DO THIS, BUT I DID *THINK* ABOUT IT.

MARISA, WHEN YOU WISH HARM ON SOMEONE, WHO ARE YOU REALLY HURTING?

OUCH, THIS THING IS KILLING ME.

YOUR AURA IS ALMOST BLACK.

I DON'T WANT TO HEAR IT, MA.

YOUR HANDS WERE MEANT TO CREATE.

SURROUND YOURSELF WITH THE LIGHT OF THE HOLY SPIRIT.

GET RID OF THE NEGATIVITY, HON.

YEAH, YEAH, YEAH, YEAH... I GOTTA GO.

MAYBE MY AURA WASN'T RADIATING POSITIVITY...

YOU'RE LOOKING A LITTLE BURNT...

...AND I DON'T GET IT, BECAUSE I'VE KNOWN YOU FOR 20 YEARS AND YOU'VE *NEVER* BEEN SO IN LOVE...

AD MOGUL RICHARD, ANOTHER BFF

TELL SHARON TO MAKE YOU A BLONDE, PUT ON BIG SUNGLASSES, GET SOME BIG HOOPS...
I THINK YOU SHOULD LOOK LIKE AN ITALIAN FILM STAR!

HE'S AN EXPERT IN PACKAGING.

LATER, I MET UP WITH LISA...

CHANGE THE MOVIE OF YOUR LIFE. COME WITH ME TO KABBALAH.

ALL I WANT IS TO CHANGE MY HAIRCOLOR.

BUT MY MOVIE SEEMED TO HAVE A LIFE OF ITS OWN, AND I WAS REALLY LUCKY...

CUE NINO ROTA, COMPOSER, WHO SCORED ALL THE GREAT FELLINI FILMS...

LIGHTS DOWN, CAMERA ON, LET'S ROLL PICTURE...

LA DOLCE VITA SILVANO STYLE

OOOOH...

AHHHH...

FLIGHT #645 FROM NEWARK TO MILAN

NO, WE'RE NOT MEMBERS OF THE MILE HIGH CLUB,

WHITE TRUFFLE ON YOUR AIRPLANE PASTA?

YOU EVEN SMUGGLED THE SHAVER ON BOARD!

IT'S BECAUSE WHEREVER YOU GO, HE WHIPS UP A GOURMET MEAL.

SHOULD I NAVIGATE FROM MILAN TO FLORENCE?

FLORENCE? LET'S GO RIGHT TO ST. TROPEZ!

HE'S ALWAYS UP (FOR 24 HOURS STRAIGHT, 9 HOURS IN THE AIR, 15 IN THE CAR) FOR AN ADVENTURE.

SILVANO, YOU REALLY KNOW HOW TO LIVE.

TANKS. I DO IT EVERY DAY!

THE GLASS IS NEVER HALF EMPTY.

YOU KNOW SOMETING... BEFORE, YOU WERE TOO TIN.

TANKS.

HE IS SO ITALIAN.

AND IT HAS ME WORRIED—

—STOP TINKING! YOU TINK TOO MUCH! AHH...CHE BELLA GIORNATA!

ON THE EXACT DATE OF THE DAY I WILL NEVER FORGET AS LONG AS I LIVE...

AT THE EXACT MOMENT OF...

...ME, B.C., LEFT FOREVER, NEVER TO RETURN TO ANSWER...

KNOCK, KNOCK.

APT C

WHO'S THERE?

CANCER.

CANCER WHO?

SMASH!

CANCER YOUR WEDDING! CANCER YOUR CAREER! CANCER YOUR LIFE!

WAS IT SOMETHING I SAID?
WAS IT SOMETHING I ATE, DRANK, SMOKED, INHALED,
PUT ON, PUT INSIDE MY BODY?
WHY? WHY? WHY? WHY IS THIS HAPPENING
NOW, JUST WHEN I'M ABOUT TO GO TO
CITY HALL IN 3 WEEKS TO GET MARRIED
FOR THE FIRST TIME AT 43...
AT 43...HELLO UP THERE...

THIS IS *KIND* OF
A BIG MOMENT FOR ME...

INSTEAD OF
SHOPPING FOR
A WEDDING
GOWN...

...I'M SEEING
MYSELF IN
A HOSPITAL
GOWN.

AND NOW, BACK TO THE WORST MOMENT I'VE EVER HAD IN ALL OF MY 43 YEARS, BACK TO WHERE I TOLD...

SILVANO, THE GOOD NEWS IS WE CAUGHT IT EARLY...

IT'S OK, I'M 'ERE. YOU'LL BE FINE.

BUT THERE'S SOMETHING ELSE I HAVE TO TELL YOU...

THIS IS THE HARD PART...

WHAT ELSE IS THERE?

I HOPE THIS DOESN'T DESTROY US.

ACTUAL ELAPSED TIME: 4.5 SECONDS. BUT IT FELT LIKE 4.5 LIFETIMES.

FIRST I HAVE TO TELL YOU THAT...

I LOVE YOU MORE THAN LIFE ITSELF.

OOH. IF ONLY THAT TV TREATMENT HAD GONE INTO DEVELOPMENT, I WOULDN'T BE IN THIS MESS...

IN SICKNESS AND STUPIDITY...

... MY INSURANCE RAN OUT.

I'M UNINSURED.

MY LIFE IS OFFICIALLY OVER.

BUT WHY DIDN'T YOU TELL ME WHEN I ASKED YOU IF YOU 'AD IT?

66

SO SILVANO WENT BACK TO WORK...

AND I TRIED TO GET BACK TO WORK...

I THOUGHT I COULD WORK THROUGH ANYTHING...

...ng Mom and Dad

Treo

SILVANO IS THE GREATEST MAN IN THE WORLD.

WE DIDN'T DOUBT HIM FOR A MINUTE...AND WE'RE HERE TO HELP, TOO,...IF YOU WANT TO SPEAK TO YOUR MOM, SHE'S WHERE ELSE,...

I'M ON THE PHONE, HON. YOUR DAD GAVE ME AN ENEMA SO I COULD POOP.

UGH...THANKS FOR THE MENTAL IMAGE, MOM.

THEN I PHONED MY GAL PALS AND GAVE THEM THE SENSATIONAL SCOOP.

KIMBERLEY...≥SOB≤ ...I HAVE TO...

ANNE...≥SOB≤ ≥SOB≤...HAVE A...

SALT WATER FISH

ALEX...≥SOB≤ ...LUMPECTOMY. ≥SOB≤ ≥SOB≤ ≥SOB≤

I NEED A LITTLE AIR.

SO I LEFT OUR PLACE AND HEADED TO THE OLD BACHELORETTE PAD. WE KEPT IT FOR STORAGE, AND VISITING RELATIVES FROM ITALY. BESIDES. NEW YORK REAL ESTATE IS IMPOSSIBLE TO COME BY...

IT WAS LIKE WALKING INTO A TIME CAPSULE OF MY FORMER SELF.

PILES OF IDEAS

THE PLACE WAS STILL A FIRE HAZARD

MY CLOSET WAS STILL PACKED WITH SUPER SKINNY SIZE Os.

THOSE DAYS WERE LONG GONE

HERE'S WHERE I STARTED TO...

SNAP!

YOU!!!!

THIS IS ALL BECAUSE OF YOU!!!!

HAD SHE BEEN ALIVE, MY GRANDMOTHER WOULD BE SHATTERED; THIS VANITY WAS HER FAVORITE PIECE.

SMASH!

EXHAUSTED, I CRASHED IN MY OLD BED.

I SAW MARY ON MY LEFT...

SHE SEEMED SAD AND PEACEFUL

...WHICH WAS IRONIC BECAUSE SHE WAS STEPPING ON A SNAKE SHE SLAUGHTERED.

FIERCE.

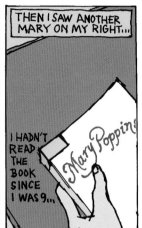

THEN I SAW ANOTHER MARY ON MY RIGHT...

I HADN'T READ THE BOOK SINCE I WAS 9...

Mary Poppins

...AND I REALIZED BEFORE SHE WAS *DISNEYED* INTO SWEET MARY POPPINS...

MARY WAS KIND OF A BITCH!

HUMPH!

KIND OF A BITCH?!

THE PITY PARTY'S OVER, C'MON GET UP...

SPIT-SPOT!

ZZZZZZT

YOU'LL NEVER CONQUER ANYTHING BY LYING IN BED ALL DAY.

WHY IS THIS HAPPENING TO ME?

RING! RING!

HELLO?

MARISA, LISA. THERE ARE 2 THINGS WE NEED TO DO. FIRST I'M TAKING YOU TO SEPHORA.

BUT I DON'T WANT TO GET A LIPSTICK.

THEN COME TO THE KABBALAH CENTRE; THEY'RE DOING A HEALING TONIGHT.

I DON'T WANT TO GO THERE, EITHER.

C'MON, YOU'LL GET THE LIGHT!

N.
O.
NO.

OFFICIAL WALLOWING TIME 5 HOURS, 37 MINUTES

RING! RING!

YOU HAVE TO TALK TO LINDA THALER, SHE'S A BREAST CANCER SURVIVOR AND AN INSPIRATION.

RICHARD WAS IN FULL CEO MODE ON THE WEEKEND

ONE OF MY DEAR FRIENDS JUST MARRIED AN ONCOLOGIST AT MEMORIAL SLOAN-KETTERING; AND YOU HAVE TO SEE HIM!

FASHION EXECUTRIX ANNIE CRACKING THE WHIP

YOU HAVE TO EDUCATE YOURSELF; I'LL GO ONLINE AND SEND YOU SOME RESEARCH.

MY COUSIN LINDA IS A DENTIST

I JUST FOUND THE TOP ONCOLOGIST IN THE WORLD... YOU HAVE TO GO TO HER!

SHARON'S CLIENTS WERE THE MOST POWERFUL WOMEN IN NY

YOU HAVE TO GET A 2ND OPINION, I'D GET A 3RD, 4TH, 5TH, 6TH, 7TH, 8TH...

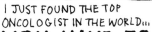

YOU HAVE TO GO TO THE HEALTH FOOD STORE AND GET MAITAKE MUSHROOM SUPPLEMENTS—IT FIGHTS TUMORS!

ALEX WAS A REDHEAD THAT WEEK

IT'S KIMBERLEY; MY UNCLE ANTHONY IS A DOCTOR AT ST. VINCENTS, YOU HAVE TO TALK TO HIM!

73

WHEN SILVANO CALLED, I FINALLY GOT OUT OF BED AND WENT HOME.

OH, IT'S LATE. I GOTTA GO.

WHERE ARE YOU GOING?

KABBALAH.

KABBALAH?!

RELAX. YOU'RE MARRYING A CATHOLIC.

7:02. OUTSIDE THE KABBALAH CENTRE...

SHABBAT SHALOM.

SHABBAT SHALOM. BY THE WAY, YOUR PAL RIVAL CARTOON GIRL MIGHT BE HERE.

WHAT?!?!

SHE'S THE LAST PERSON I WANT TO SEE. YOU KNOW HOW MUCH I H—

SHH! WE'RE TRYING TO MAKE YOU HEALTHY!

..YOU'RE HERE TO GET THE TOOLS TO HELP YOU TRANSFORM...

...AND BREAK YOUR DESTRUCTIVE HABITS.

INSIDE THE KABBALAH CENTRE:

DURING SHABBAT, THE MEN WEAR ALL WHITE AND YARMULKES. EVEN GUY RITCHIE WEARS A YARMULKE.

WHY DO THE WOMEN HAVE THE SAME HAIR?

THEY'RE WIGS; MARRIED WOMEN WEAR THEM.

THE WIGS WERE STYLED BY THE SAME HAIRSTYLIST. IS THAT SOMETHING I'D HAVE TO THINK ABOUT?

LISA, I FEEL OUT OF PLACE...

I DON'T KNOW...

75

THE SERVICE WAS ABOUT TO BEGIN, SO WE MADE OUR WAY TO THE PEW. (I DIDN'T KNOW WHAT ELSE TO CALL THEM.)

WE "SCANNED" THE HEBREW LETTERS AS EVERYONE SANG...

ידיד נפש אב הרחמן,

...AND "DOWNLOADED" THE ENERGY... READ RIGHT TO LEFT

משוך עבדך אל רצונך,

retz'onecha el avdecha meshoch

ירוץ עבדך כמו איל

a'val k'mo avd'cha yarutz

...TO MAKE THE "CONNECTION" TO THE LIGHT.

THEN THEY SHUT THE LIGHTS OFF AND SANG SONGS OF HEALING...

...AND THAT'S WHEN IT HAPPENED.

...I HAD THE SENSATION THAT AN ANTENNA CAME OUT OF THE KABBALAH CENTRE...

...BROADCASTING LIGHT FROM THE CITY...

...TO THE ENTIRE COUNTRY...

...THE WHOLE WORLD...

I SAW FACES... ...PLACES... PEOPLE I DIDN'T KNOW... ...PEOPLE I DID KNOW... AND LOVE...

...AND IN THAT MOMENT I FELT A CONNECTION TO HUMANITY... AND AN OVERWHELMING SENSE OF PEACE.

THEY SAY THE EARTH IS IN THE SUBURBS OF THE PINWHEEL OF THE GALAXY.

WHEN THE LIGHTS WERE TURNED ON, I TOLD LISA...

YOU HAVE TO TELL MEIR, MY KABBALAH TEACHER. C'MON LET'S HAVE DINNER. THE FOOD IS 5 STAR OF DAVID.

I'LL STAY A BIT, BUT I'M HAVING DINNER WITH SILVANO.

AS THEY ATE, I TOLD MEIR WHAT I "SAW," AND HE DIDN'T BLINK AN EYE.

YOU ARE AN ANTENNA OF LIGHT.

WE ALL ARE.

10:37. I WAS 7 MINUTES LATE AND ABOUT TO TURN INTO A PUMPKIN...

HOLY SPIRIT, PLEASE PUT WHITE PROTECTIVE LIGHT AROUND SILVANO AND ME.

MARISA, 'URRY UP. I WANT TO EAT NOW. OH THERE YOU ARE, I WAS JUST CALLING YOU!

DaSilvano

AT 11:19, WHEN WE FINALLY SAT DOWN, I LOOKED ACROSS THE TABLE AND THOUGHT ABOUT HOW HAPPY I WAS WITH SILVANO...

AHH... PERFECT, I MADE THIS FOR YOU.

HOW HAPPY I WAS TO BE ALIVE...

WE BOTH HAD SPAGHETTI AL POMODORO

TOMATOES ARE AN EXCELLENT SOURCE OF THE CANCER-FIGHTING LYCOPENE, FYI.

IT WAS THE BEST PASTA I EVER HAD, AND I SAVORED EACH AND EVERY BITE LIKE IT WAS MY LAST.

AS WE WERE FINISHING DINNER, CLAUDIO, SILVANO'S BFF, JOINED US. HE WAS IN FROM ITALY DOING SOME BUSINESS IN THE STATES.

CIAO, SILVANO!

CIAO, MARISA!

SILVANO TOLD ME. I'M VERY SORRY.

IT'S OK, CLAUDIO, I'M LOOKING AT IT LIKE IT'S AN OPPORTUNITY.

AN OPPORTUNITY?!!

BO. *

* "BO" MEANS "I DON'T KNOW."

WHAT I MEAN IS, INSTEAD OF SEEING THE TUMOR AS A BLACK HOLE...

...I'M LOOKING AT IT AS A WHITE PEARL OF OPPORTUNITY TO CLEAN EVERYTHING UP AND GET RID OF MY TOXIC BEHAVIOR.

AND THAT'S ALL THAT HAPPENED ON MAY 15, 2004, THE DAY THAT WILL BE FOREVER KNOWN TO ME AS "D. DAY," AKA "DIAGNOSIS DAY"...

I'M EXHAUSTED.

ME TOO.

AN OPPORTUNITY?

THE NEXT DAY, WE TOOK A SPIN IN SILVANO'S ITALIAN SPORTS CAR...

CHE BELLA GIORNATA!

IT /S A BEAUTIFUL DAY!

RING! RING!

T Mobile

Dina Calling

IT'S MY SISTER.

HI, DINA.

I WISH IT WERE ME!

DINA, DON'T WISH IT ON ANYONE...

ESPECIALLY YOURSELF.

I'M FINE.

WHY IS IT YOU?!

I DON'T KNOW...

...NOBODY KNOWS...

PLEASE STOP CRYING!

THIS WAS THE CALL THAT BROKE MY HEART.

STOP CRYING... ≷SOB!≷

PLEASE ≷SOB!≷ STOP CRYING...

STOP CRYING ≷SOB!≷

I'LL GO PARK THE CAR.

PUT THE COVER ON THE CAR AFTER IT COOLS OFF...

THIS IS FOR YOU.

PARK

ARE YOU OK?

I'M FINE.

RING! RING!

THIS IS YOUR COUSIN; I JUST TALKED TO MY FRIEND'S BROTHER'S GIRLFRIEND WHO'S A FREELANCER LIKE YOU AND SHE HAD BREAST CANCER BUT SHE DIDN'T HAVE INSURANCE...

IF HER DOCTORS HAD BILLED HER, IT WOULD HAVE COST HER $200,000!

$200,000?!?

CALL HER TOMORROW AFTER 12. SHE'S ON DEADLINE.

BO.

HER TREATMENTS COST $200,000!!!

IT'S OK... I TOLD YOU I'LL WORK IT OUT.

THE NEXT MORNING, I RANG BREAST SURGEON DR. MILLS, AND BEGAN THE ENDLESS PHONE CALLS OF MY NEW LIFE.

DR. MILLS'S OFFICE...

...PLEASE HANG ON WHILE I PUT YOU ON HOLD...

CLICK!

HA HA HA HA...STAYIN' ALIVE, STAYIN' ALIVE...

I'M NOT MAKING THIS TONY MANERO MOMENT UP.

80

THEN I WENT TO CLEAN UP MY OLD APARTMENT. MY (S)MOTHER WAS STAYING OVER.

WHAT A MESS.

I SAT DOWN AT MY OLD DRAWING BOARD AND CALLED MY COUSIN'S BEST FRIEND'S BROTHER'S GIRLFRIEND...

I'LL HOOK YOU UP WITH MY DOCTORS, I DIDN'T PAY A CENT! HOW BIG IS YOUR TUMOR?

PEN POISED FOR NOTE-TAKING ACTION

THE* TUMOR IS 1.3 CM; I'M LUCKY I CAUGHT IT EARLY.

MY TUMOR WAS 1.1 CM; I CAUGHT IT EARLY, TOO...

*I NEVER USED "MY" IN FRONT OF TUMOR. I DIDN'T WANT TO OWN IT.

...AND I HAD A DOUBLE MASTECTOMY AND I LOST ALL MY HAIR!

≥GASP!≤ I'M SORRY TO HEAR THAT...

ARE YOU OK?

WHAT ABOUT ME?!?!?!

I'M MORE THAN OK... NOW I'VE GOT THE GREATEST TITS!

HI, HON!

AWW... WHAT'S THE MATTER?

I JUST ≥SOB≤ TALKED TO THE GIRL WHO DIDN'T HAVE ≥SOB≤ INSURANCE AND SHE LOST ALL HER HAIR AND HAD A DOUBLE MASTECTOMY!

BUT YOU CAUGHT YOURS EARLY.

THE TUMOR ≥GASP!≤ SHE HAD ≥GASP!≤ WAS SMALLER ≥GASP!≤

DON'T BE AFRAID, YOU KNOW WHAT I ALWAYS SAY...

MA, DON'T SAY IT...

I ALWAYS SAY...

PLEASE, NOT TODAY...

FEAR IS THE WORK OF THE DEVIL.

BY THE WAY, YOUR GRANDMOTHER TOLD ME ABOUT THE VANITY, AND NEITHER OF US ARE UPSET.

THAT MAKES ME FEEL BETTER.

AT THE KABBALAH CENTRE, I HAD A SESSION WITH RABBI MEIR.

YEAH, YOU'RE A GOOD PERSON, BUT YOU COULD BE A BETTER PERSON.

HOW?

MEIR WAS OK WITH ME TAPING HIM.

YOU CAN SMILE.

SMILE?

MEIR...

HAVE YOU BEEN TALKING TO MY MOTHER?

MY MOTHER WAS IN THE LOBBY, ARMED WITH CATHOLIC ARTILLERY.

MOM, COME IN!

BIOGRAPHY OF A SAINT

SAINT TERESA

IN HER RIGHT HAND, HER PADRE PIO NOVENA, ON HER LEFT, HER CORD OF SAINT PHILOMENA.

WHAT DO CANCER CELLS THRIVE IN?

CHAOS.

WHAT IS CHAOS?

FEAR.

HE WAS TALKING ABOUT "CANCER CONSCIOUSNESS."

FEAR IS THE BIGGEST TOOL OF SAY-TON.

YOU SAY SAY-TON AND I SAY DEVIL.

AFTER THAT, WE WENT TO DR. MILLS FOR A CONSULTATION.

DR. MILLS, I JUST TALKED TO SOMEONE WHO HAD A TUMOR THAT WAS 1.1 CM, AND SHE HAD A DOUBLE MASTECTOMY!

SHE WAS HYSTERICAL WHEN I PICKED HER UP.

WE WERE BOTH IN FETAL POSITION.

THAT'S WHY I'M MIXED ON SUPPORT GROUPS. EVERY CANCER IS DIFFERENT.

I'M DOING A BIOPSY SO WE CAN DETERMINE WHETHER THE CANCER HAS EXTENDED THROUGH THE DUCT, AND I'M SENDING YOU FOR A MAMMOGRAM. I THINK IT'S STAGE 1 CANCER. YOU'RE *LUCKY* YOU CAUGHT IT *EARLY*.

THANK GOD I'M FLATCHESTED!

GOD? YOU SHOULD THANK *ME* FOR THAT!

THAT NIGHT, I REVISED MY PRAYERS BEFORE I SAW MY *FIDANZATO*.

PLEASE, HOLY SPIRIT, HELP ME FIND THE WORDS.

MARISA, YOU ALWAYS HAVE THE BEST SHOES. WHO MAKES THEM?

DOORMAN WITH A SHOE FETISH

THANKS, THEY'RE CESARE PACIOTTI.

EVERYTING OK?

EVERYTING'S FINE. I JUST NEED MORE TESTS.

ALTHOUGH WE MADE SMALL TALK...

CANCER CANCER

WHAT SHOULD WE EAT?

WHATEVER YOU WANT.

...I KNEW SILVANO WAS PUTTING ON A BRAVE FACE FOR MY SAKE, BECAUSE HE TOLD HIS STAFF.

CIAO, MARISA!

MARIE, 'OW ARE YOU?

ARE YOU ALRIGHT?

TUTTO BENE?

IS THERE ANYTHING I CAN GET YOU?

MAYBE SOMETHING SPECIAL THIS EVENING?

THE NEXT MORNING I JOURNEYED TO THE CENTER OF THE CARTOON UNIVERSE.

YOU'RE EARLY, KIDDO!

SAM, I NEED TO TALK TO YOU.

THE NEW YORKER EDITORIAL IS ON THE 21ST FLOOR.

OH GOD, OH NO. ISABELLE SAID "THERE IS SOMETHING VERY WRONG WITH MARISA." YOU GO SEE MANKOFF, I'LL TAKE CARE OF IT.

ISABELLE IS SAM'S WIFE, AND I LOVED HER.

HELLO!

BOB, I CAN'T STAY AND YOU'LL SEE WHY.

OOOOOO...

AND WHEN I LEFT BOB'S OFFICE...

NO CUTTING!

FIRST COME!

FIRST SERVE!

I WAS NEXT!

WHY'D YOU JUMP THE LINE?!

I'M SORRY, I HAVE BREAST CANCER, AND I HAVE TO RUN TO GET A MAMMOGRAM.

I TRIED TO TELL THEM.

84

11:45. NAZ MET ME AT THE RADIOLOGY PLACE.

YOU DON'T HAVE INSURANCE?

I'M PAYING BY CHECK.

WHY DON'T YOU HAVE INSURANCE?!

LOOK, I ALREADY FEEL BAD, DON'T MAKE ME FEEL WORSE, OK?

MARISA?

SEE YA AFTER TORTURE.

SO I HAD MY FIRST MAMMOGRAM AT 43...

AND I GOT SQUEEZED...

...SQUISHED...

...SLAMMED...

...AND JAMMED...

WHY DON'T THEY PUT *TESTICLES* IN A VISE?!

THAT AFTERNOON, I WENT BACK TO WORK WHEN...

IT'S DR. MILLS'S OFFICE; HE WANTS YOU TO COME IN AT 9 A.M. FOR A BIOPSY.

I CALLED MY (S)MOTHER, WHO INSISTED ON COMING TO EVERYTHING...

THAT MEANS I HAVE TO GET UP AT 5 A.M., LEAVE AT 6 A.M. TO GET THERE AT 8:30 TO PICK YOU UP. NO, 9 A.M. DOESN'T WORK FOR ME.

THE POT STIRRER

YOU WANT ME TO ASK DR. MILLS TO ARRANGE HIS HEAD OF THE HOSPITAL SURGEON'S SCHEDULE AROUND HIS PATIENT'S MOTHER?!

THEN I RANG DR. MILLS'S OFFICE, AND HE GOT ON THE PHONE...

NO! I NEED YOU HERE AT 9 A.M., TIME IS OF THE ESSENCE!

BELIEVE IT OR NOT, NEXT I HEARD FROM A DOCTOR'S WIFE...

HI MARISA, ANNIE MARINO GAVE ME YOUR NUMBER. MY HUSBAND IS A DOCTOR AT SLOAN-KETTERING.

THANKS, BUT I DON'T HAVE INSURANCE AND MY DOCTORS AT ST. VINCENTS ARE HELPING ME OUT.

I DIDN'T KNOW IT THEN, BUT THIS IS WHEN MY FRIENDS BEGAN CONSPIRING...

SHE SAID *WHAT*?! NOW WE HAVE TO DEAL WITH THIS BECAUSE SHE IS NOT DEALING!

AT THE END OF THE NIGHT, AFTER THE A-LISTERS LEFT AND THE PAPARAZZI PACKED IT IN FOR THE EVENING, I WAITED FOR SILVANO TO CLOSE UP SHOP...

LET'S GIVE THIS TO THE MTA WORKERS BEFORE WE GO, C'MON.

'EY GUYS, 'OW ABOUT SOME ESPRESSO?

THANK YOU, MR. SILVANO.

WOW, THAT'S SOME GOOD COFFEE.

WE NEED IT TO STAY AWAKE.

...AND THEN THE NIGHT CREW WENT DOWN TO WORK ON THE 6TH AVENUE SUBWAY LINE.

GOODNIGHT!

THE NEXT MORNING...

I'M IN THE TUNNEL!

IT'S YOUR MUDDER.

IT'S 7 A.M.! I TOLD HER IT WOULD ONLY TAKE 30 MINUTES TO GET HERE!

7:21. I MET MY (S)MOTHER IN THE LOBBY.

I GOT A POST FOR YOU AND A POST FOR SILVANO. GO BACK AND GIVE IT TO HIM.

NO. YOU'VE ALREADY WOKEN HIM UP ONCE.

MOM, WHAT'S WITH THE NECK BRACE?

DON'T WORRY ABOUT YOUR POOR MOM.

AILMENT #1: SCIATICA

7:37, GREY DOG. THE MOST LAID BACK COFFEE SHOP IN LOWER MANHATTAN...

WILL YOU LOWER YOUR VOICE? THAT GIRL IS LISTENING TO EVERY WORD!

BREAKFAST #1: (S)MOTHER HAD OATMEAL. I HAD COFFEE.

WE HAVE TO TALK TO DR. MILLS ABOUT THE FACT THAT YOU DON'T HAVE INSURANCE—

PLEASE. MOM. BE QUIET. THIS IS THE 2ND TIME I ASKED.

I DON'T WANT THE WORLD TO KNOW ABOUT MY EPIC SCREWUP!

I DON'T GIVE AN EFF-ING—

SLAM!

REFILL #3

THAT'S IT! GO HOME! YOU AND YOUR BIG FAT MOUTH GO BACK TO NEW JERSEY!

YOU'RE UPSETTING ME! YOU'RE NOT HELPING ME!

87

I'M THE ONE WITH CANCER HERE!

BUT WE STILL HAVE TO DEAL WITH THE FACT THAT YOU HAVE NO INSURANCE!

C'MON, LET'S GO TO CHURCH.

WHY, SO I CAN TELL GOD TO GO TO HELL?

OUR LADY OF POMPEII CH

1 ROSARY AND 3 NOVENAS LATER...

I'M AFRAID TO SAY ANYTHING RIGHT NOW.

OH, THAT'S A FIRST.

8:12. ROCCO'S PASTRY.

WHAT ARE YOU HAVING?

BREAKFAST #2: MOM: DECAF CAPPUCCINO AND A BRIOCHE, ME: CAPPUCCINO AND A PANETTONE, WHICH MY (S)MOTHER ATE.

8:32. WE WERE FINALLY ON OUR WAY TO DR. MILLS'S OFFICE.

I'M SORRY I'M SORRY I'M SORRY I'M SORRY—

YOU KNOW, THEY CAN HEAR YOU UP THERE.

BEFORE THE DREADED CORE BIOPSY, DR. MILLS FILLS US IN.

CANCER
LUMPECTOMY
MAY NOT BE INVASIVE
LYMPH NODES.

THE LAST DOCTOR'S VISIT WITHOUT A TAPE RECORDER.

9:32. DR. MILLS BIOPSIED ME BY STICKING A NEEDLE IN THE TUMOR, THEN YANKING OUT THE SLIVERS OF CANCER.

I FEEL REALLY FAINT.

SIT DOWN. I'LL GET YOUR MOM.

NEEDLE #2:

ACTUAL WIDTH

4" ACTUAL LENGTH

THE CORE BIOPSY NEEDLE IS WIDER THAN THE THIN ASPIRATOR NEEDLE, AND IT IS MORE ACCURATE BECAUSE IT TAKES OUT MORE CELLS.

ACTUAL SIZE OF THE BIOPSIED WORMY BASTARDS

MARISA

YOU MAY HAVE CAPTURED US, BUT THERE'S A MILLION MORE WHERE WE CAME FROM.

10:18. ANGLERS & WRITERS.

THANKS, MOM. I NEEDED TO EAT.

THIS IS RUINING MY WEIGHT WATCHERS.

RING! RING!

BREAKFAST #3: ME: WESTERN OMELETTE, HASH BROWNS, BACON, COFFEE. (S)MOTHER: PANCAKES & COFFEE.

I GOT A CALL FROM A FRIEND WHO SHALL REMAIN NAMELESS...

MARISA, YOU DIDN'T CALL THE "IT" ONCOLOGIST, THEY CALLED ME! HE'S KEEPING HIS OFFICE OPEN ON MONDAY SO YOU CAN GET YOUR SECOND OPINION, AND FOR YOUR SAKE YOU BETTER BE THERE!

CLICK!

OOF, YOUR FRIENDS ARE SO BOSSY!

BOSSINESS IS LOVE, AND YOU'RE THE C.E.O. OF BOSSY.

89

MARISA, SILVANO. I WANTED TO KNOW 'OW YOU'RE FEELING?

I'M A LITTLE WIPED, BUT I FEEL OK.

LISTEN, I GOT INVITED TO COOK FOR A PARTY ON LABOR DAY WEEKEND. THEY WERE GOING TO FLY US OUT BY 'ELICOPTER TO THEIR 'OUSE IN SOUTH 'AMPTON.

I WAS TINKING YOU MAY NEED A CHANGE OF SCENERY?

THAT SOUNDS GREAT, BUT I THINK I MAY BE HAVING SURGERY.

OK, I'LL LET THEM KNOW THAT I'LL LET THEM KNOW, CIAO- I-LOVE-YOU.

CLICK!

RING! RING!

palmOne

T-Mobile

Dr. Mills calling

THIS IS DR. MILLS'S OFFICE. YOU'RE SCHEDULED FOR SURGERY MAY 26.

MAY 26? HANG ON, LET ME CHECK...

...THAT MORNING I'VE GOT A BROW WAXING FOLLOWED BY A MEETING UPTOWN, THEN LUNCH WITH AN EDITOR; IN FACT AS I LOOK AT MY CALENDAR I SEE THE WHOLE MONTH IS COMPLETELY BOOKED. SO, I'M SORRY...

...BUT WE'LL HAVE TO DO THAT LUMPECTOMY AT ANOTHER TIME WHEN IT'S MORE CONVENIENT FOR ME...

CIAO!

IF I SAID THAT, I WOULD NEED TO GET MY HEAD EXAMINED, ON TOP OF EVERYTHING ELSE.

HERE'S WHAT I REALLY SAID...

MAY 26...?!

27, 28, 29, 30, 31 1, 2, 3, 4, 5, 6, 7, 8, 9, 10, 11= 16 DAYS... HMM...

WILL I BE OK BY JUNE 11?!

SURGERIES ARE LIKE WEDDINGS: THEY'RE ONLY REAL WHEN YOU'VE SET A DATE.

I NEED TO TAKE A NAP.

11 MINUTES LATER:

RING! RING!

I SLEPT ON MY BACK BECAUSE OF THE BIOPSY ↓

MARISA, IT'S MATT... ARE YOU SURE YOU'RE UP FOR DOING "THE REJECTION SHOW" TONIGHT?

OF COURSE I'M UP FOR IT; BESIDES, MATT... I PROMISED YOU I'D DO IT!

OUCH!

AND I THOUGHT IT WOULD BE GOOD FOR ME.

I CAREFULLY GOT READY, CONSCIOUS OF THE BANDAGES...

OUCH!
OOH!
OW WWW!

GRANDMA'S SEQUINED SHIRT. SHE MADE IT HERSELF IN THE '50s. →

'ALLO, 'ALLO! I'M 'OME... YOU'RE GOING OUT?!

I'M DOING "THE REJECTION SHOW," REMEMBER?

CHE É "THE REJECTION SHOW"?

IT'S A SHOW WHERE WRITERS, COMEDIANS, CARTOONISTS, ANYONE PERFORMS THEIR REJECTED MATERIAL TO A LIVE AUDIENCE ONSTAGE.

AND YOU'RE DOING THIS TODAY?!

YEP. SEE YA AT 10:30. I LOVE YOU. CIAO!

HI. 42ND BETWEEN 9TH AND 10TH, PLEASE.

RING! RING!

REESE, IT'S ANNIE. WHAT'S GOING ON WITH THE SECOND OPINION?

I'M AFRAID WHINE WHINE NO INSURANCE WHINE WHINE WHINE WHAT SHOULD I SAY? WHINE WHINE HELPING ME OUT WHINE SIMPER AM I A WIMP? WHIMPER WHIMPER—

I'LL CALL YOUR DOCTOR, WHAT'S HIS NUMBER?

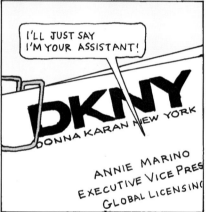

I'LL JUST SAY I'M YOUR ASSISTANT!

DKNY
DONNA KARAN NEW YORK

ANNIE MARINO
EXECUTIVE VICE PRES
GLOBAL LICENSING

3 MINUTES LATER:

NO BIG DEAL. THEY *EXPECT* YOU TO GET A SECOND OPINION.

NOW YOU JUST HAVE TO FAX A LETTER TO RELEASE YOUR MATERIALS, OK?

BUT I STILL THINK YOU SHOULD GO TO SLOAN!

OH LORD, EVERYONE HAS A MILLION OPINIONS AND I DON'T HAVE ONE.

TAXI

EXCUSE ME, MISS?

REMEMBER MY PILES OF REJECTS?
WELL, *NEW YORKER* CARTOONIST MATT DIFFEE
INGENIOUSLY FOUND SOMETHING FOR
THE REST OF US CARTOONISTS TO DO WITH THEM...

THE
REJECTION
SHOW

SOLD OUT

HI, I'M THE REJECTED CARTOONIST.

NO CHARGE FOR PERFORMERS.

TICKETS $10.00

MATT COCREATED "THE REJECTION SHOW"...

LET'S GO ONSTAGE AND DO A RUN-THROUGH. I EDITED YOUR BATCH DOWN TO 10.

GREAT EDIT, BY THE WAY.

HERE'S YOUR CHANCE TO PROVE YOUR STUFF IS FUNNY, IF THE AUDIENCE LAUGHS. FIRST I'LL INTRODUCE YOU AND YOU'LL PUT A CARTOON ON THE PROJECTOR...

...THEN IT'LL BE PROJECTED ON THE SCREEN HERE, AND WE'LL TELL STORIES OF OUR LIVES AS CARTOONISTS... WE'LL TAKE TURNS.

YOU MEAN OUR LIVES OF REJECTION. YOU KNOW, SAM ONCE SAID THAT THE AVERAGE DISAPPROVAL RATING FOR A CARTOONIST IS 97%. THAT MEANS 3% OF OUR STUFF IS PRINTED.

BEFORE THE SHOW STARTED, I WAITED AT THE BAR AS MY FRIENDS CAME IN...*

JUST HAVE FUN WITH THIS THING, KIDDO.

SAM, I LOVE THAT YOU CALL ME KIDDO AT 43.

* I SENT OUT A MASS E-MAIL, AND I GOT A GOOD RETURN.

I ALSO E-MAILED MY COUSIN'S BEST FRIEND'S BROTHER'S GIRLFRIEND, SHE OF THE 1.1-CM TUMOR, DOUBLE MASTECTOMY, COMPLETE HAIR LOSS FAME...

MARISA?

HILARY, I THOUGHT THAT WAS YOU...

... BECAUSE OF YOUR TITS!

SHH!

SHE GAVE ME A LOT OF POSITIVE POINTERS.

I'M A SWIMMER AND I SWAM THROUGH ALL OF MY TREATMENTS.

I SWIM 5 TIMES A WEEK, WILL I KEEP DOING THAT?

YOU TWO, TAKE IT SOMEWHERE ELSE!

95

COME ON, LET'S GO TALK IN THE GREEN ROOM.

AND I'M A WRITER AND I NEVER MISSED A DEADLINE.

WAIT, LET ME INTRODUCE YOU TO MY FIANCÉ.

HI, I'M BRETT AND I KNOW YOUR COUSIN BRUNO.

HI BRETT, NICE TO MEET YOU.

BRETT, GIVE US A FEW MINUTES.

YOU KNOW, I'M ENGAGED, TOO.

YOU'RE ENGAGED? HERE'S WHAT HAPPENED TO ME AND IT'S GONNA HAPPEN TO YOU...

WHAT?!

HE'S NEVER GOING TO MARRY YOU!

HI, I'M MATT DIFFEE, NEW YORKER CARTOONIST, AND I'M PLEASED TO INTRODUCE MY FELLOW CARTOONIST... MARISA ACOCELLA!

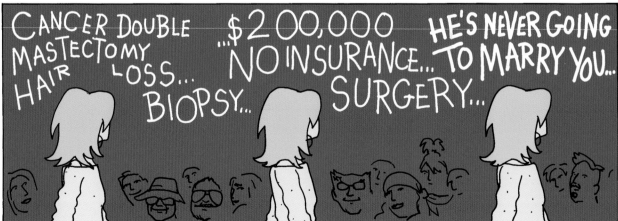

CANCER DOUBLE MASTECTOMY HAIR LOSS... BIOPSY... $200,000 ...NO INSURANCE... SURGERY... HE'S NEVER GOING TO MARRY YOU...

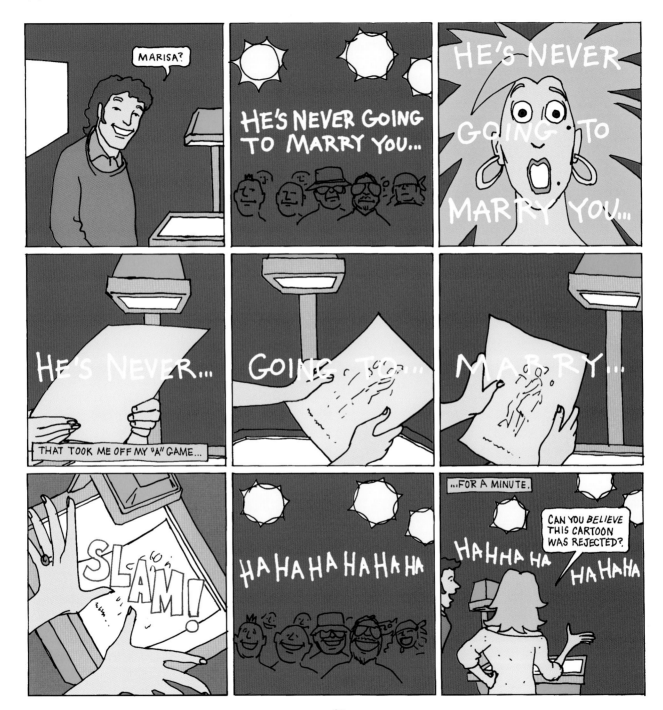

Panel 1:
HERE'S THE UPSIDE OF TELLING PEOPLE YOU'VE BEEN DIAGNOSED. YOU TELL A FRIEND...

Panel 2:
THEN THEY TELL THEIR FRIENDS...

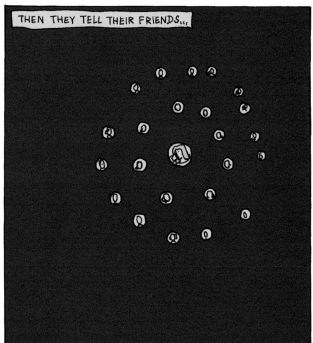

Panel 3:
AND SO ON...

...AND SO ON...

...AND YOU'VE CREATED YOUR OWN SUPPORT UNIVERSE.

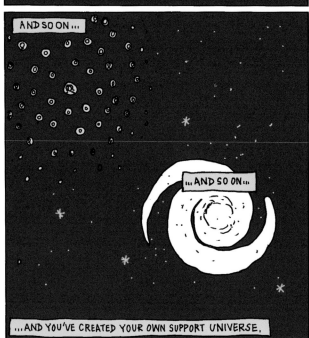

Panel 4:
ME, B.C., WAS SO FOCUSED ON THE ENVY AND HATRED AROUND ME, I LOST SIGHT OF ALL THE LOVE.

I KNOW WE'RE NOT BEST FRIENDS, BUT I'LL GO WITH YOU TO WHATEVER.

HOW ARE YOU?

MY MOTHER HAD IT, TOO. IS THERE ANYTHING I CAN DO?

I READ ABOUT THIS SALVE.

I CAN DO YOUR CHART.

THESE WERE PEOPLE I BARELY KNEW...

BUT THERE IS A DOWNSIDE...

RIGHT AFTER THE REJECTION SHOW, I SWUNG BY THE RESTAURANT...

THE SHOW WAS GREAT, THANKS.

VERY GOOD. I NEED A FEW MINUTES.

THEN WAITED AT OUR TABLE, WHICH WAS NEXT TO TOM AND NAZ.

YOU MISSED IT. SOME GIRL GAVE SILVANO HER NUMBER, AND HE FED HER CARD TO A DOG!

HE DID NOT.

YES HE DID, THAT DOG OVER THERE!

SO, HOW'S YOUR CANCER?

DO I EVEN KNOW YOU?

UGH! CAN YOU BELIEVE HER?

IGNORE HER.

I'LL BELIEVE ANYTHING.

2 HALF PORTIONS OF PASTA WITH FRESH JALAPEÑO LATER...

SILVANOOO...

HERE'S MY CARD...

I'M NOT SICK...

...CALL ME IF YOU WANT A HEALTHY RELATIONSHIP.

MY FRIENDS CALL THESE TATTOOS "ASSLERS"

'ERE, BOY...

MANGIA!

WHAT THAT WOMAN SAID WAS *THE* MOST DESPICABLE...

I'M TRYING TO LET IT GO...

OH C'MON, STOP TINKING ABOUT IT!

FLASH! FLASH! FLASH! FLASH!

PAPARAZZI SHOOTING STARS

WHEN I TOLD MY GAL PALS...

OK, I WOULD HAVE DUMPED A BOWL OF PUTTANESCA ON HER HEAD.

SO WHAT IF *THAT* WAS REPORTED!

PRINT HER NAME!

THERE'S A SPECIAL PLACE IN HELL FOR BITCHES LIKE THAT.

ANNIE

LISA

PAULA IS NEWLY SINGLE, HMM...

AND AFTER I GOT PAST THAT CHEESY NEW AGE MUSIC ON THE PSYCHIC HOTLINE, SOMEWHERE IN MONTANA...

HE'S MARRYING YOU EVEN AFTER YOU HAD CANCER *AND* HE'S MAKING SURE YOU GET INSURANCE...

BUT I GOTTA TELL YA POINT-BLANK, I WOULDA TAKEN OUT MY 12-GAUGE AND ASKED HER TO LEAVE.

DR. NIKKI NAMED HER WINCHESTER 1300 "PREDATOR"

HER HUSBAND, REVEREND JIM, CALLS HIS BY ITS NAME: "DEFENDER"

DR. NIKKI HAS DOCTORATES IN DIVINITY AND THEOLOGY.

THE NEXT MORNING:

I WOKE UP

STIPPLED,

LOOKING LIKE

A MANKOFF CARTOON.

I NEED TO SEE THE DOCTOR ASAP!

MARISA, IT'S THAT TIME OF THE MONTH AGAIN!

GLAMOUR IS ON THE 16TH FLOOR OF THE CONDÉ NAST BUILDING

WHAT'S GOING ON IN YOUR LIFE RIGHT NOW?

FUNNY YOU SHOULD ASK....

NYU Medical Center

BREAST CANCER? I'M SO SORRY....

LAUREN BRODY, MY GLAMOUR EDITOR

DO YOU WANT TO WRITE ABOUT IT?

MOMENTS LATER, I ENTERED THE OFFICE OF DERMATOLOGIST DR. BRUCE STROBER.

No Cellular Phones

OFF!!

IT'S ECZEMA. HAVE YOU BEEN UNDER A LOT OF STRESS LATELY?

OH, JUST THE USUAL WORK STRESS, BRIDAL STRESS, BREAST CANCER STRESS.

NYU HOSPITAL GOWN WITH THE SIDE TIE IS VERY "DVF"—DIANE VON FURSTENBERG

I'M SORRY. MY WIFE IS A PSYCHIATRIST AT SLOAN. IF THERE'S ANYTHING I CAN DO, LET ME KNOW.

THANKS, DOCTOR.

101

IN THE MEANTIME, THESE MOLES ON YOUR FACE CAN BE JUST AS BAD...

IF THEY'RE CANCER.

CANCER?!

BLACK HOLES CONSUME AT GREAT SPEED...

NOT AGAIN!

WHAT IT DECIDES TO DEVOUR IS RANDOM, JUST LIKE WHO GETS CANCER AND WHO DOESN'T IS A MYSTERY.

LUCKILY, I WAS NO BLACK HOLE SNACK.

YOU LOST ME THERE FOR A MOMENT.

CAN I DO A BIOPSY?

I CAN'T TAKE ANOTHER BIOPSY!

I DON'T HAVE INSURANCE! THIS IS JUST TOO MUCH!

I HAVE TO DOCUMENT IT. YOU'RE OK NOW, BUT WE HAVE TO MONITOR IT FOR YOUR HEALTH.

DR. STROBER ALMOST HAD HIS BACK TO ME. A BORDERLINE BAD SIGN.

No ar Phones

RING! RING!

Lauren calling

HEY, LAUREN.

I JUST TALKED TO CINDI AND SHE *LOVES* THIS IDEA...

CINDI LEIVE IS THE EDITOR IN CHIEF.

7R Dermatol

...AND WE ALL SAY "ANYTHING BAD THAT HAPPENS TO YOU IS REALLY GOOD MATERIAL"!!

DR. GOLDSTEIN HAD ASKED ME TO GET CHEST X-RAYS, SO I WENT BACK TO WHERE I HAD THE MAMMOGRAM...

IF YOU DON'T HAVE INSURANCE, YOU HAVE TO PAY UP FRONT.

OK, HOW MUCH DO I OWE YOU?

AFTER THE CHEST X-RAY...

DR. GOLDSTEIN, WHY DID I HAVE A CHEST X-RAY?

WE WANTED TO MAKE SURE YOUR CHEST IS CLEAR—

·MY CHEST IS CLEAR OF WHAT?!

THE POSSIBILITY OF SKIN CANCER AND NOW *LUNG* CANCER ON TOP OF BREAST CANCER WAS TOO MUCH FOR ME TO DEAL WITH...

MISS, ARE YOU OK?

AFTER THAT, I HAD ANOTHER SESSION WITH RABBI MEIR...

The Kabbalah Centre

YOU COME HERE FOR A PURPOSE...

YOU GET THE BEST HAIR, AND THEN WHAT?

YOU GET THE BEST BAG, AND THEN WHAT?

I KNOW...

THE BEST SHOES!

DUMB JOKE.

WHAT'S THE PURPOSE?

THE HEBREW ALPHABET HAS NUMERICAL VALUE...

EVERY LETTER HAS A NUMBER, AND YOU CAN ADD THE NUMBERS UP IN EACH WORD...

LOOK, MARISA...

...THAT'S THE MISSION OF THE HUMAN RACE...

אהבה
(LOVE = 13)

אחד
(ONE = 13)

...TO LOVE AS ONE AND BE AS ONE.

START FROM LOVING YOURSELF.

IT'S BOB AND I'M BACK FROM IBIZA. I GUESS EVERYTHING'S OK BECAUSE I HAVEN'T HEARD FROM YOU... RIGHT?

I JUST DIDN'T WANT TO RUIN YOUR TRIP...

HUDSON RIVER PARK, 26 MINUTES LATER:

THIS WILL CHEER YOU UP: DID YOU READ THE *BEAUTIFULLY* DETAILED BLOW-BY-BLOW ACCOUNT OF OUR *FAVORITE* LIT GIRL GETTING AN ASS-KICKING—

—BOB, NO NEGATIVITY, OK?

I'M STUDYING KABBALAH.

ALL THIS BAD ENERGY AROUND ME HAS TAKEN ITS TOLL.

WELL, I AM *NOT* GOING TO SUGGEST THAT CANCER WAS BROUGHT ON BY YOUR TOXICITY!

PEOPLE WHO DO THAT MAKE ME NUTS.

RIGHT NOW I'M NOT DISCOUNTING ANYTHING.

INSTEAD OF CHANGING YOUR MINDSET, CHANGE THAT OUTFIT! SWEATPANTS? SNEAKERS? YOU'RE THE DAUGHTER OF A SHOE DESIGNER! YOU LOOK LIKE A VICTIM...

WHERE'S MY VIXEN?

BUT I'M TOO DEPRESSED TO RUN AROUND IN 5-INCH HEELS GOING FROM "IT" EVENT TO "IT" EVENT! WHO CARES?

YOU DON'T HAVE TO SHOW UP FOR THEM. BE THERE FOR YOURSELF. *YOU'RE* MORE *IMPORTANT* NOW...

YOU'RE RIGHT, I DON'T HAVE TO DO THE THINGS I DON'T WANT TO DO, AND IN A WEIRD WAY... NOW I HAVE THE POWER TO SAY NO.

INTRODUCING THE CANCER CARD

WHEN YOU CARRY THE CANCER CARD, IT GETS YOU OUT OF DINNERS, LUNCHES, BREAKFASTS, BRUNCHES, SOCIAL OBLIGATIONS, FAMILY FUNCTIONS, CONCERTS, SHOWS, SPORTING EVENTS, PARTIES, MOVIES AND MORE!

ENJOY THE CANCER CARD EASY-ACCESS BENEFITS!
NO LICENSE?
NO PHOTO I.D.?
NO PROBLEM!

NO PRESET SPENDING LIMIT—YOUR CARD IS THERE WHEN YOU NEED IT! INSTANT APPROVAL! UNIVERSAL SURVIVOR NETWORK—NOW THAT YOU'RE A MEMBER, HOTLINE OTHER SURVIVORS WHO CAN ASSIST YOU ON PHYSICIANS, MEDICATIONS AND MORE!

A SPECIAL KIND OF MEMBERSHIP.

MAY 24. 1 P.M. MY (S)MOTHER AND I WENT UPTOWN TO "IT" ONCOLOGIST, DR. NATURAL, THAT MY NAMELESS FRIEND INSISTED I SEE...

I'M WILLING TO EXPLORE ANYTHING, BUT I DON'T KNOW WHAT TO THINK ABOUT A HOLISTIC CANCER TREATMENT.

HE BETTER BE A MIRACLE DOCTOR FOR THE AMOUNT OF MONEY HE'S CHARGING.

WE WAITED IN HIS RECEPTION AREA.

I EXPECTED THIS PLACE TO BE CLEAN AS A WHISTLE.

HEY MARISA, ISN'T HE SUPPOSED TO BE DR. NATURAL?

YEAH, WHY?

WELL, DR. NATURAL HAS ARTIFICIAL PLANTS.

AS WE CONTINUED WAITING, I DID SOME CARTOONS. BESIDES, I WAS ON DEADLINE, AS USUAL.

WHAT DO YOU THINK OF THIS?

HMM...

I'M HAVING A BAD WIG DAY.

WHEN AT THAT MOMENT...

DAPHNE, WHEN DOES THE DOCTOR WANT TO SEE YOU AGAIN?

IT'S DIFFERENT WHEN YOU SEE IT.

GASP!—

FINALLY, AFTER 2 HOURS...

MARISA, COME ON IN.

DR. "IT" AKA NATURAL WORE MEPHISTOS

WHILE IN HIS OFFICE, WE LISTENED AS HE GAVE HIS HOLISTIC LECTURE...

THAT WAS FLY NUMBER 5.

MEPHISTO IS ANOTHER NAME FOR SAY-TON.

...AND AS HE TOLD US HE RECOMMENDS SOY AND GREEN TEA.

WRONG. SOY ACTS LIKE ESTROGEN AND COULD ACCELERATE TUMOR GROWTH, AND GREEN TEA MAY OXIDATE CANCER CELLS DURING CHEMO.

I DIDN'T KNOW IT THEN, BUT I CERTAINLY KNOW IT NOW.

NEEDLE #3

HE TOOK ME INTO HIS EXAMINING ROOM WHERE HE DREW BLOOD, AND THEN...

HE TOLD ME TO LIE DOWN AND RELAX AND LISTEN TO THE SELF-MADE MEDITATION TAPE THAT HAD HIS OWN VOICE-OVER.

THIS MUSIC SOUNDS FAMILIAR.

WHAT IS IT...?

WAIT, IS IT...?

OH I CANNOT BELIEVE IT!

IT WAS ANYTHING BUT RELAXING.

AS I WAS LEAVING THEY GAVE ME HIS PRESS KIT, BOOKS HE HAD WRITTEN AND THE MEDITATION TAPE.

THANKS?

MOM, I SPENT A HALF HOUR LISTENING TO THE CHEESY NEW AGE MUSIC FROM THE PSYCHIC HOTLINE!

YOU'RE GONNA NEED A SECOND OPINION AFTER YOUR SECOND OPINION.

PFFT... ARTIFICIAL PLANTS!

Panel 1: 4:05. WE HEADED BACK DOWNTOWN FOR A 5:00 WITH GENERAL PRACTITIONER DR. PAUL GOLDSTEIN.

ORGANIC

I'M HUNGRY. SHOULD WE EAT VEGAN?

I'D FEEL LIKE A CANCER PATIENT.

ORGANIC & MACROBIOTIC

Panel 2: 4:20. JOE JR.'S COFFEE SHOP.

I'M HAVING YOU BROTHER DAVID'S FAVORITE.

WHAT'S THAT?

Panel 3: BACON TOMATO AND CREAM CHEESE ON A BAGEL

IT DISAPPEARED IN 5 SECONDS FLAT. OK, I EXAGGERATED, 59 SECONDS.

Panel 4: MA, WHATEVER YOU DO, DON'T SAY ANYTHING ABOUT THAT DOCTOR.

MY DAUGHTER SAID NOT TO SAY ANYTHING, HELLO!

Panel 5: I MEAN IT. I WANT TO MAKE MY OWN DECISION.

$600 A VISIT AND $350 FOR A BLOOD TEST YOU DIDN'T EVEN ASK FOR.

Panel 6: MOM, I NEED TO MAKE UP MY OWN MIND, OK?

HE *WAS* HIGHLY RECOMMENDED.

MARISA, COME ON IN.

NEEDLE #4

THE BLOOD-DRAWING NEEDLE #2 THAT SAME DAY.

Panel 7: SPEAKING OF DRAWING...

MAYBE I CAN SKETCH WITH MY FEET TONIGHT?

Panel 8: HELLO, DOCTOR. I'M MARISA'S MOM.

OH, SHE LOOKS LIKE YOUR SISTER!

Panel 9: YOUR CHEST X-RAYS ARE CLEAR.*

EXCUSE ME, MAY I SAY SOMETHING?

*THAT'S GOOD NEWS, I DON'T HAVE *LUNG* CANCER.

111

THAT NIGHT I GOT A CALL. NOPE. THIS ISN'T MY MOM...

MARISA...

PADRE PIO

I'M PREGNANT!

ARE YOU ON, TOO, VIOLETTA? I HAVE TO THANK YOU FOR THE CORD OF ST. PHILOMENA, I EVEN SHOWERED WITH IT ON!

WHILE SHARON, WHO'S JEWISH, WORE THE CORD OF A CATHOLIC SAINT...

SHARON, YOU'RE PREGNANT!

...CATHOLIC ME WAS STUDYING JEWISH MYSTICISM KABBALAH.

SAINT PHILOMENA IS SO POWERFUL.

THIS WAS THE HAPPIEST OF MOMENTS

THE NEXT MORNING, I WENT ONLINE TO READ ABOUT BREAST CANCER.

TAP! TAP! TAP! TAP!

BREAST CANCER IS THE SECOND LEADING CAUSE OF CANCER-RELATED DEATH IN WOMEN

AFTER THAT, I WENT TO MY THERAPIST. I WAS GOING UNDER THE KNIFE IN LESS THAN 24 HOURS!

YOU'RE WHAT'S IMPORTANT...

YOU NEED TO FEEL ENTITLED TO YOUR NEEDS...

WHAT WERE YOU JUST THINKING OF?

THIS IS WHAT I WAS THINKING OF, AND IT WAS THE MOST SATISFYING CHEESEBURGER DELUXE I EVER HAD.

IT WAS MY FAVORITE MEAL AS A KID. MAYBE I WAS CRAVING A TIME WHEN I WAS COMPLETELY CAREFREE?

JOHNNY ROCKETS
THE ORIGINAL HAMBURGER
42nd East 6th St
New York, New York 10003

05/25/2004
2:17 PM

Server: Kadir
2/1
Guests: 1   #10066

                              2.09
                              1.59
American Fries   0.59
Original
  Add Cheddar-Tillamook   7.07
                              0.61

Sub Total
Tax   7.86

Total   7.68

Balance Due

FREE HAMBURGER w/ purchase of
hamburger, starter and drink.
Call 1-800-

Survey Validation Code:_____
Redeem one per 3 month period

How long will I be in the hospital?

What kind of anesthesia am I getting?

How will my normal routine be restricted?

How much discomfort will I have?

What kind of bandages will I have after surgery?

How should I care for the bandages after surgery?

When do I get the bandages off?

Will I have a scar?

How many lymph nodes are you taking out?

What are my chances of developing lymphedema?

Are there any side effects from surgery?

When should I come back for a follow-up visit?

What kind of care will I need after surgery?

How soon can I go back to my regular schedule?

Does Saint Vincents take Amex?

Or can I write a check?

DR. MILLS, I HAVE A QUESTION. DON'T YOU THINK SHE SHOULD COME HOME TO NEW JERSEY SO I CAN TAKE CARE OF HER?

I'LL BE OK I'LL BE OK DON'T WORRY I'LL BE OK.

EVEN THOUGH SHE PROBABLY WON'T STAY OVERNIGHT... THIS IS A MAJOR PROCEDURE...

TRANSLATION: THERE WILL BE PAIN.

YOU'LL NEED SOMEONE TO TAKE CARE OF YOU.

HER (S)MOTHER!

TRANSLATION: YOU WILL FEEL AND LOOK LIKE HELL.

THAT AFTERNOON I GOT CALLS FROM WELL-WISHERS...

IT'S KIMBERLEY...

IT'S SAM...

IT'S ANNE...

IT'S ALEX...

IT'S LEYLA...

IT'S KIRSCH...

IT'S LINDA...

IT'S DINA...

IT'S YOUR BROTHER...

DAD'S ON THE LINE.

AND WOULD YOU BELIEVE THAT VERY DAY WAS THE FEAST OF SAINT PHILOMENA. A SPECIAL MASS WAS SAID FOR ME BY FATHER DON GIOVANNA, AND SISTER BERTILLA PLACED MY PICTURE ON THE ALTAR.

SAINT PHILOMENA'S BONES ARE ENTOMBED IN PAPIER MÂCHÉ WITH A BEAUTIFUL ROBE AND DISPLAYED IN A GLASS CASE

SHE'S THE PATRON SAINT OF WOMEN AND THOSE WHO ARE IN DANGER

I AM HERE

SANCTUARY OF SANTA PHILOMENA, AVELINO, ITALY

I'M AN ATHEIST AND I'M PRAYING FOR YOU.

THAT'S NOT TRUE, RICHARD. YOU'RE A PROTESTANT!

THAT EVENING, AFTER AN EARLYISH DINNER AT 10...*

SILVANO, DON'T TAKE THIS THE WRONG WAY, BUT I'D PREFER IT IF YOU DIDN'T COME TO ST. VINCENTS...

SINCE I WAS HAVING GENERAL ANESTHESIA THE NEXT MORNING I COULDN'T EAT OR DRINK PAST MIDNIGHT.

I KNOW IT'S RIDICULOUS, BUT I ONLY WANT YOU TO SEE ME AT MY BEST...

BESIDES, MY MOM WANTS TO GO AND HER FAVORITE SOAP IS GENERAL HOSPITAL.

SO WE WENT HOME AND...

MIND IF I DISROBE?

...THIS IS EXACTLY WHAT I WAS AFRAID OF, ESPECIALLY SINCE I WAS GETTING MARRIED IN 17 DAYS.

6:45 A.M. SURGERY DAY.

CIAO, I LOVE YOU. I LOVE YOU, CIAO.

COME ON WE CAN'T BE LATE!

THIS WAS GOING TO BE OUR FIRST NIGHT APART SINCE MAY 2002.

DID YOU REMEMBER TO WEAR A BUTTON DOWN SHIRT, HON?

AFTER THE SURGERY, I WOULDN'T BE ABLE TO LIFT MY SHIRT OVER MY HEAD.

7:01. ST. VINCENTS HOSPITAL. BEFORE SURGERY, I NEEDED TO HAVE "THE INJECTION."

THANK GOD I STAYED OVER IN YOUR OLD APARTMENT. TUNNEL TRAFFIC WOULD HAVE BEEN A KILLER.

MOM, WHAT'S WRONG WITH YOUR HANDS?

AILMENT #2: CARPAL TUNNEL SYNDROME.

7:23, THEY GAVE ME A ROBE, SLIPPERS, MY VERY OWN GARMENT BAG AND A FEW OTHER GOODIES...

THE BEDPAN IS THERE IN CASE YOU VOMIT.

I'LL HOLD YOUR HEAD IF YOU THROW UP.

I FORGOT MY LENS CASE, SO I PUT MY CONTACTS IN THE CONTAINERS THEY USE FOR URINE SAMPLES.

SIT UP STRAIGHT, I'LL GO GET THE PAPER.

MISS ACOCELLA!

BEFORE YOU GO IN, I'M TYING THE CORD OF ST. PHILOMENA ON YOU.

AND DON'T LOSE THIS ONE!

THEN I GOT BRIEFED BY DR. KODE EDIALE.

YOU'RE FROM NEW JERSEY? WELL, TO GO INTO NEW YORK, BEFORE YOU GO INTO THE TUNNEL, YOU HAVE TO PAY THE TOLL...

THE TOLL IS THE SENTINEL NODE.

HOLLAND TUNNEL

...IF THE CANCER CELLS ARE IN THE LYMPH NODES, THEY WOULD REACH THE SENTINEL NODE FIRST.

TO FIND THE SENTINEL NODE, WE INJECT A RADIOACTIVE TRACE AND A BLUE DYE INTO THE BREAST. THIS WILL TRAVEL TO THE SENTINEL NODE IN THE ARMPIT AND HELP IDENTIFY IT. A GEIGER COUNTER WILL LOCATE THE SENTINEL NODE.

BTW, DR. EDIALE LOOKED LIKE MY GRANDFATHER

AFTER WE DO THE LUMPECTOMY WE'LL REMOVE THE SENTINEL NODE AND DO A "FROZEN SECTION" TO SEE IF IT'S POSITIVE OR NEGATIVE.

ARE WE THERE YET?

THIS IS THE "FACES) PAIN INTENSITY SCALE"...

ON A SCALE OF 1 TO 10, THE PAIN OF THE INJECTION IS A 7...

I COULD GIVE YOU A CREAM TO NUMB THE AREA, BUT I'M NOT SURE IT WORKS.

2   4   SEVERE PAIN   6   8   VERY SEVERE PAIN   10   WORST POSSIBLE PAIN

MARISA ACOCELLA

NEEDLE #5

THE RADIOACTIVE TRACER

OOOOOOO HHHHMY GOD!!!

THE NEEDLE WENT IN THE AREA BEHIND THE NIPPLE, WHERE THERE ARE A LOT OF SENSORY FIBERS

OUCH.

MY GOD IS A WOMAN

FOR THE RECORD, THE PAIN WAS OFF THE CHART

IT GOES TO "11"

10   ME →

SPEAKING OF TOLLS, I HAD TO PAY THE BILL UP FRONT BEFORE GOING INTO SURGERY...

BILLING

HERE'S WHAT HAPPENS WHEN YOU DON'T HAVE INSURANCE...

PEOPLE GO IN AND OUT AND YOU'RE STUCK THERE FILLING OUT FORM AFTER FORM, THEN FINALLY YOU PAY BY CARD AND WAIT FOR IT TO BE PROCESSED.

YOUR FATHER AND I ARE PAYING FOR IT, HON.

THANK YOU.

FINALLY, AFTER AN HOUR, YOU BUST OUT OF BILLING, STRESSED AND TRYING TO FIND SURGERY...

THAT WAY?

NO, THAT WAY!

YOU FIND YOUR SURGEON WAITING FOR YOU BECAUSE HE HAS ALL THE TIME IN THE WORLD ON HIS HANDS.

♪ whistling ♪

AND THE OPERATING ROOM IS BACKED UP FOR THE REST OF THE DAY BECAUSE THEY HELD IT FOR YOU.

WHAT MARVELOUS CONDITIONS TO GO UNDER THE KNIFE!

11:11, I WAS GIVEN A GENERAL AND WAS ON THE OPERATING TABLE...

OK, WE'RE GOING TO EXCISE THE TUMOR AND...

...I WAS OUT.

3:15-ISH.

THE OPERATION WAS A SUCCESS, AND IT LOOKS LIKE THE MARGINS WERE CLEAR.

IF THE TUMOR WAS LIKE A PEACH PIT, THERE WERE NO FUZZY CANCER TENTACLES ON THE PERIMETER.

AND IT ALSO LOOKED TO THE DOCTORS LIKE IT DIDN'T SPREAD INTO MY LYMPH NODES... PHEW!

CANCER

6 P.M. MY PARENTS' HOUSE IN NEW JERSEY, I WAS SURROUNDED BY MY FAMILY...

MY BROTHER ANTHONY

MY SISTER DINA

AUNTIE RISA, HOW ARE YOU?

MY NEPHEW, JOHNNY

MY ICED BREAST

...AND MY COUSINS.

I PADDED MY BREAST BECAUSE I DIDN'T WANT YOU TO FEEL ALONE.

MY COUSIN LINDA THE DENTIST

TOTAL # OF CALLS: 27
TOTAL # OF CALLS FROM SILVANO: 21

119

VROOM!

9:32 A.M.

QUICK, WASH YOUR FACE.

THAT COULD ONLY BE ONE SOUND!

9:33 A.M.

"EY, I BET YOU THOUGHT I ABANDONED YOU.

WELL...WATCH THE BOOB.

I THOUGHT YOU FELL ASLEEP, SO I DIDN'T CALL, BUT I'M 'ERE NOW.

LET'S BRING YOUR BAG UPSTAIRS.

SILVANO'S FANCY ITALIAN SPORTS CAR

STRADALE

9:34 A.M.

EXCUSE US, THIS IS A PRIVATE MOMENT, BUT I WILL SAY I'VE NEVER FELT MORE LOVED IN MY LIFE.

THEN WE UNPACKED THE TRUNK...

WHAT DID YOU DO? BRING THE WHOLE RESTAURANT?

WHO'S THE CEO OF THE CEO OF BOSSY?

VIOLETTA, CAN YOU PLEASE CHOP THE GARLIC?

WHATEVER YOU SAY, SILVANO.

AT NOON, WE ALL SAT DOWN AND DEVOURED FAGIOLI ALL' UCCELLETTO...

AHH, PERFECT....

THAT'S CANNELLINI BEANS IN TOMATO SAUCE.

THIS IS THE FIRST TING I'VE EATEN SINCE WEDNESDAY.

I'VE NEVER KNOWN HIM TO MISS A MEAL.

I'M SO SORRY YOU'RE GOING THROUGH THIS.

OH, IT'S OK.

BUT IT'S NOT ME, IT'S YOU WHO I'M WORRIED ABOUT.

122

JUNE 3. (8 DAYS FROM OUR WEDDING!)
I HAD MY FIRST POST-OP VISIT WITH DR. MILLS,
WHERE WE DISCUSSED MY NEXT STEPS...

Patient: **ACOCELLA, MARISA**
Med Rec: **V1191439**

Location: CANCER CENTER
Physician: CHRISTOPHER MILLS, MD

Case: **VVS-04-7184**
Reg #: V000440830719
Procedure Date: 05/26/2004
Date Received: 05/26/2004
Date Reported: 05/29/2004

Chris mills
5/30/04

SURGICAL PATHOLOGY REPORT

SPECIMEN: A: BREAST, WITH MARGINS, left, lumpectomy. **B:** LYMPH NODE, SENTINEL, left axillary, #1 hot and blue. **C:** LYMPH NODE, SENTINEL, left axillary adjacent node.

FINAL DIAGNOSIS:

PERFORMED AT SAINT VINCENTS COMPREHENSIVE CANCER CENTER
325 WEST 15TH STREET, NEW YORK, NY 10011

A- <u>LEFT BREAST LUMPECTOMY:</u>
- **INFILTRATING MODERATELY DIFFERENTIATED DUCTAL ADENOCARCINOMA, NOS, 1.3X1.1 CM**, WITH PROMINENT DESMOPLASTIC REACTION
- THE INVASIVE CARCINOMA SHOWS HIGH HISTOLOGIC GRADE (3/3), INTERMEDIATE NUCLEAR GRADE (2/3), AND INTERMEDIATE MITOTIC COUNT (2/3). SBR SCORE: 7/9, GRADE II
- **RARE FOCI OF DUCTAL CARCINOMA IN SITU (DCIS)**, SOLID TYPE, NON-COMEDO WITH CENTRAL NECROSIS, INTERMEDIATE NUCLEAR GRADE (2/3) INVOLVING ISOLATED DUCTS WITHIN THE INVASIVE TUMOR
- ONE FOCUS SUGGESTIVE OF

YOU HAD EARLY BREAST CANCER. THE TUMOR IS COMPLETELY REMOVED. IT WAS 1.3 CENTIMETERS.

CHEMOTHERAPY AND HORMONE THERAPY ARE SYSTEMIC TREATMENTS. THEY TREAT THE WHOLE BODY. THEY LESSEN THE RISK OF THE DISEASE SPREADING SOMEWHERE ELSE.

SURGERY AND RADIATION ARE LOCAL TREATMENTS.

RADIATION TREATMENT TO THE BREAST SIGNIFICANTLY REDUCES THE RISK OF RECURRENCE. RADIATION IS GIVEN BECAUSE THERE COULD BE CELLS IN TRANSIT THAT HAVE BEEN UNDETECTED.

CAN'T YOU GO ANY FASTER?

NEGATIVE FOR MALIGNANCY, 0/1
- CYTOKERATIN STAIN AE-1/AE-3 IS NEGATIVE FOR MALIGNANT CELLS

C- <u>LEFT AXILLA, ADJACENT LYMPH NODE:</u>

When can I get the bandages off?

Can I use my arm?

What kind of exercises should I be doing?

What kind of exercise should I not be doing?

What stage of cancer did I have?

How would you define it?

Did the cancer jump anywhere else in my body?

Is there a chance that some cells are wandering in my body that haven't been detected?

What are my next steps?

Why do I need chemo?

SO, ON DR. MILLS'S RECOMMENDATION, I CALLED FOR AN APPOINTMENT WITH DR. PAULA KLEIN, A MEDICAL ONCOLOGIST AT ST. VINCENTS COMPREHENSIVE CANCER CENTER (SVCCC)...

WHAT'S YOUR INSURANCE?

IT WAS FOR JUNE 29 AT 1:30.

THEN I CALLED FOR AN APPOINTMENT WITH DR. JOHN RESCIGNO, A RADIATION ONCOLOGIST AT SVCCC.

WHAT'S YOUR INSURANCE?

NO APPOINTMENT SET YET.

DR. MILLS, I JUST GOT THE RUNAROUND.

MARISA, DON'T WORRY... I'LL TAKE CARE OF IT.

WHEN I TOLD MY FRIENDS THE SENSATIONAL CHEMO NEWS...

RICHARD SAID: "GET A FABULOUS WIG, BABE... IN PINK!"

KIMBERLEY SAID: "I'LL BUY YOU SOME PUCCI SCARVES, YOU'LL BE SO CHIC!"

LISA SAID: "LET'S GO HAT SHOPPING."

THIS HAT LOOKS LIKE LISA

SHARON SAID: "BUY A WIG NOW, GET YOUR HAIRSTYLIST TO MATCH YOUR HAIR, THEN I'LL COLOR IT AND NOBODY WILL KNOW IT'S A WIG!"

CAN THEY MATCH MY WIDOW'S PEAK AND COWLICKS, TOO?

I SAID:

"HEY, I'M AN ARTIST. I NEVER MET A SURFACE I DIDN'T LIKE!"

ON AN UP NOTE, I GOT A CALL FROM BOB AT *THE NEW YORKER*

YOU GOT AN "OK"... AND I ALSO WANTED TO KNOW HOW YOU'RE DOING.

R. MANKOFF

FOR THE RECORD, HIS ASSISTANT CALLS 99% OF THE TIME WHENEVER WE SELL A CARTOON.

THAT NIGHT, WHEN I SAT DOWN WITH SILVANO...

JUST AS WE THOUGHT, MY DOCTORS FEEL I NEED CHEMO...

...IT'LL IMPROVE THE ODDS OF THE CANCER NOT COMING BACK.

ALL RIGHT, YOU'LL BE OK...

I WASN'T SURPRISED BY HIS REACTION...

CAN WE LEAVE NOW? WE 'AVE TO GET UP EARLY AND GET OUR MARRIAGE LICENSE!

...HE ALWAYS FOCUSES ON THE POSITIVE.

JUNE 11. THIS 43-YEAR-OLD AND HER YOUNG-AT-HEART FIDANZATO TOOK THAT TRIP TO CITY HALL...

ARTHUR SMARSCH, OUR DETECTIVE PAL, DROVE US IN AN UNMARKED CAR. THE CITY WAS ON A "RED" TERROR ALERT THAT DAY.

SAY "PARMIGIANO," MR. AND MRS. MARCHETTO!

OUR WITNESSES WERE LEYLA, THE RING BEARER,

MY MOM AND DAD.

THE GROOM WORE ORANGE LEATHER

WE WERE "WEDDING OF THE WEEK" IN THE NEW YORK POST

PHOTO BY VIOLETTA ACOCELLA

AFTER OUR WEDDING, WE DROVE TO MONTREAL FOR THE WEEKEND TO SEE THE GRAND PRIX...

CIAO! CIAO!

ARRIVEDERCI, SIGNORE E SIGNORA!

BUON VIAGGIO!

JUST MARRIED

STRADA

SEE YA!

WE WEREN'T GOING ON OUR HONEYMOON JUST YET. I NEEDED TO MEET WITH ONCOLOGISTS FIRST.

AT THE GRAND PRIX, A MIRACLE HAPPENED. SILVANO, MY HUSBAND, THE MAN WITH MORE ENERGY THAN ANYONE, THE MAN WHO IS IN PERPETUAL MOTION AND HAS NEVER WASTED A PRECIOUS SECOND ON THIS PLANET, SAT STILL WITHOUT MOVING AN INCH FOR 2 SOLID HOURS AND WATCHED AS HIS FAVORITE DRIVER, MICHAEL SCHUMACHER, WON

THIS MAY SOUND CRAZY, BUT WHEN I SAW THAT 1,000,000-WATT SMILE OF HIS LIGHT UP AFTER ALL WE'D BEEN THROUGH...

...IT WAS THE SINGLE MOST HAPPIEST MOMENT OF MY LIFE, AND IT'S NOT JUST BECAUSE I LOVE FORMULA 1, TOO.

WE CAME BACK FROM OUR MINI-HONEYMOON AND MY FRIENDS...

CONGRATULATIONS TO YOU BOTH!

AND THEN...

NOW MARISA, WHAT ABOUT THE SECOND OPINION?

I'M AFRAID THAT IF I GO TO MEMORIAL SLOAN-KETTERING, THAT MEANS I HAVE SERIOUS CANCER.

ARE YOU INSANE?!

WE KNOW YOU HAVE FAITH IN ST. VINCENTS...

BUT YOU DON'T HAVE TO GO TO THE SAME HOSPITAL FOR YOUR TREATMENT.

IF YOU'RE NOT TAKING CANCER SERIOUSLY, ARE YOU IN DENIAL?!?

CAN YOU TELL THEY LOVE ME?

DID SOMEBODY SAY THEY KNEW SOMEONE SOMEWHERE AT SLOAN?

MY FRIEND'S HUSBAND IS AN ONCOLOGIST AT SLOAN, YOU JERK! YOU TALKED TO HIS WIFE AND YOU TOLD HER YOU WERE WORRIED ABOUT INSURANCE!

I DID.

NOW I CAN GO BACK TO RESEARCHING WIGS.

NOT UNTIL YOU MAKE ME BLONDER!

FRIDAY JUNE 18, 10 A.M. OUR SUITCASES WERE PACKED. I LEFT MY CANCER BAGGAGE BEHIND BECAUSE I WAS GOING ON A CANCER VACATION.

RING! RING!

WHERE IS THAT DAMN PHONE?

SILVANO, LEYLA AND I WERE GOING TO THE FOOD AND WINE FESTIVAL IN ASPEN. WHEN YOU'RE A RESTAURATEUR, THAT'S A BUSINESS TRIP.

JUNE 22. I MET WITH RADIATION ONCOLOGIST DR. JOHN RESCIGNO.

RADIATION STARTS 2 WEEKS AFTER CHEMO.

ST. VINCENTS COMPREHENSIVE CANCER CENTER (SVCCC) IS A BRAND-NEW FACILITY

IT'S INCONVENIENT AND IT'S DAILY, 5 DAYS A WEEK FOR 6 ½ WEEKS.

SOME WOMEN GET FATIGUE, YOU'LL GET REDNESS OF THE SKIN.

HE WOULDN'T LET ME TAKE HIS PICTURE...

THE TOTAL DOSE IS STANDARDIZED TO CONTROL THIS DISEASE 95% OF THE TIME.

...BUT HE WAS OK WITH ME TAPING HIM, SO I DEALT.

WHAT ARE THE OTHER SIDE EFFECTS?

RADIATION CAN CAUSE CANCER. IN YOUR CASE IT'S 1 IN 1,000 IN 15 YEARS, AND 1 IN 500 IN 30 YEARS.

MAY I SAY SOMETHING?

IT'S LIKE TRYING TO STOP A FREIGHT TRAIN.

ALL MY FRIENDS WHO HAVE HAD CANCER, ALL THEY EAT IS CHICKEN CHICKEN CHICKEN CHICKEN CHICKEN CHICKEN CHICKEN!

CHICKEN?!

I'M TOTALLY HORMONAL!

MOO... ME TOO!

HORMONES. HORMONES. HORMONES. LIKE THE INDUSTRIAL-STRENGTH DOSAGE OF THE PILL I TOOK IN THE LATE '70s.

WHAT ABOUT RADIATION?

OR A MAMMOGRAM?

OR X-RAYS?

WHAT ABOUT THE THINGS THAT ARE SUPPOSED TO SAVE US FROM CANCER...

FAB SLINGBACKS.

HELLO, DOCTOR.

OK, BECAUSE YOU'RE STAGE-1 NODE-NEGATIVE, YOU CAN HAVE EITHER ADRIAMYCIN, "AC," THE HEAVY CHEMO, OR YOU CAN HAVE CYTOXAN, METHOTREXATE AND FLUOROURACIL, "CMF," WHICH IS THE LIGHT CHEMO.

CHEMO LIGHT. LIGHT CHEMO...

ENJOY

CHEMO LIGHT

...THAT SOUNDS LIKE A SOFT DRINK...

THERE'S NOTHING SOFT ABOUT IT... CHEMO LIGHT IS STILL CHEMO.

DR. KLEIN, LET ME BE REALLY STRAIGHT. MY HUSBAND OWNS A RESTAURANT WHERE THE MOST BEAUTIFUL WOMEN GO AND I CAN'T LOOK LIKE CRAP!

...AND I WILL KILL MYSELF IF I LOSE MY HAIR!

SHE WILL KILL HERSELF IF SHE LOSES HER HAIR.

WILL KILL HERSELF IF SHE LOSES HER HAIR.

TICK! TICK! TAP! TAP! TAP!

GOT IT.

YOU KNOW, I WOULD NEVER LET YOU RISK YOUR LIFE TO SAVE YOUR HAIR.

I KNOW. DO YOU REALLY THINK I'M LUCKY ENOUGH TO HAVE CHEMO LIGHT?

I DO, OTHERWISE I WOULDN'T SUGGEST IT IN YOUR CASE. DO YOU THINK YOU'LL BE HAVING YOUR TREATMENT HERE?

I'LL LET YOU KNOW AFTER I GO TO SLOAN.

JULY 8. MY (S)MOTHER MET ME AT THE EVELYN H. LAUDER BREAST CANCER CENTER AT MEMORIAL SLOAN-KETTERING.*

* COMPLETED IN 1992, THE FIRST-EVER BREAST AND DIAGNOSTIC CENTER WAS EQUIPPED BY A FUND INITIATED BY MRS. LAUDER.

IN OCTOBER 1992, SHE INTRODUCED NATIONAL BREAST CANCER MONTH BY DISTRIBUTING PINK RIBBONS AND BREAST SELF-EXAM CARDS, PLACING BREAST CANCER IN THE FOREFRONT OF PUBLIC AWARENESS.

IN 1993, MRS. LAUDER ESTABLISHED THE BREAST CANCER RESEARCH FOUNDATION, WHICH HAS RAISED OVER $125 MILLION.

** NONDENOMINATIONAL.

SAINT EVELYN

THE PATRON SAINT OF BREAST CANCER**

I AM IN AWE.

HOW MANY LIVES HAS SHE HELPED SAVE?

FIRST, DR. CATHERINE VON POSNIAK, MEDICAL ONCOLOGIST, EXAMINED ME.

I WOULD ALSO SEND YOU TO A DERMATOLOGIST TO LOOK ALL OVER YOUR SKIN, EVEN BETWEEN YOUR TOES, BECAUSE THERE'S A LINK BETWEEN BREAST CANCER AND MELANOMA.

BY THE WAY MSKCC IS THE WINNER! OF THE MOST GLAM GOWN HANDS DOWN!

BACK IN HER OFFICE, DR. VON POSNIAK ADVISED ME ON TREATMENT:

WITH STAGE-1 NODE-NEGATIVE, I WOULD RECOMMEND A CHEMO WHERE YOU WON'T LOSE YOUR HAIR, BUT IT COULD THIN. IT'S CALLED CMF.

THAT'S THE LIGHT CHEMO DR. PAULA KLEIN SUGGESTED.

DR. PAULA KLEIN IS AN EXCELLENT, EXCELLENT DOCTOR. BECAUSE YOU'VE SEEN ME TODAY, YOU'LL ALWAYS BE MY PATIENT, BUT YOU'RE IN GOOD HANDS WITH HER. ANYTHING ELSE?

MY HUSBAND AND I HAVEN'T HAD OUR HONEYMOON YET, DO I HAVE TIME NOW?

HMM... IT TAKES 6 TO 8 WEEKS FOR THE TISSUE TO HEAL AFTER SURGERY...

... SO GO TO ITALY NOW, THEN START YOUR TREATMENT IN 2 WEEKS.

NOW?

YOU HAVE TO LIVE YOUR LIFE!

TELL THAT TO YOUR FRIENDS.

YOU NEED TO MAKE A DECISION ASAP; THE CLOCK IS TICKING.

I THOUGHT SHE WAS BRILLIANT, MAYBE I SHOULD GO TO SLOAN?

THAT NIGHT, MY PARENTS MET ME AT DA SILVANO...

YOU LOVED DR. KLEIN. YOU LOVE DR. MILLS. DR. GOLDSTEIN IS YOUR FRIEND AND ST. VINCENTS IS DOWNTOWN.

GO WHERE YOU'LL FEEL COMFORTABLE.

JULY 9, THE NEXT DAY

HEY, PAULA, CHEMO SUCKS BUT YOU'RE GENIUS AND HILARIOUS SO MAYBE IT WON'T BE TOO TERRIBLE. BESIDES, YOU HAVE GREAT SHOES, AND I AM ON ASSIGNMENT FOR *GLAMOUR*.

CHEMO DOES SUCK. HOW LONG WILL YOU BE IN ITALY?

ANOTHER PAIR OF PAULA'S SPECTACULAR SLINGBACKS

CAN WE GO FOR 3 WEEKS?

3 WEEKS?! CALL ME FROM THE TARMAC!

OFF WE WENT ON OUR WHIRLWIND HONEYMOON IN ITALY, WHERE WE ATE AND ATE. I ENJOYED IT BECAUSE HEY, I WAS GOING TO LOSE WEIGHT ON CHEMO!

DON'T WORRY IF YOU PUT ON A FEW POUNDS.

YOU SHOULD DO A CARTOON... "THE CHEMO DIET."

LAUREN, MY *GLAMOUR* EDITOR

EAT NOW. YOU'LL FEEL TOO SICK TO EAT LATER!

BOB MANKOFF, MY *NEW YORKER* CARTOON EDITOR

EVERY DAY WAS MAGICAL IN ITALY, BUT AT NIGHT...

MY HUSBAND AND I A CUCCHIAIO. — THAT'S SPOONING IN ITALIAN

THERE I WAS DRAWING IN THE DARK ON THE EDGE OF A HIGHWAY...

SUDDENLY, I WAS ATTACKED BY AL-QAEDA???!!!

WHY AM I DRAWING IN THE DARK?!

WE'RE STILL ON THE DREAM STATE HIGHWAY...

≥ GASP! ≤

AHH... A NICE JUICY RIB EYE... RARE...

LATER THAT DAY...

IN THE NIGHTMARE, MOM, THE AL-QAEDA "CELLS" THAT ATTACKED ME ON MY OWN SOIL WERE REALLY CANCER CELLS... AND DOES IT MEAN I STILL HAVE CANCER?!

MARISA, CALM DOWN. YOUR DOCTOR SAID YOU'RE CANCER-FREE AS OF MAY 26!

BUT THERE'S A 10% RISK CELLS COULD EXIST SOMEWHERE ELSE IN MY BODY!

THAT'S WHY YOU'RE HAVING CHEMO, HON.

CHORTLE! CHORTLE! UGH GLUCK! UGH GLUCK!

THE GROSS-OUT-CLEARING-THE-THROAT-THING.

I GUESS YOU COULD SAY I WAS A TAD ANXIOUS.

DR. PAULA, I'M ON THE TARMAC. WHEN SHOULD I START TREATMENT?

135

"CUT AND HIGHLIGHT YOUR HAIR BEFORE TREATMENT, BECAUSE PULLING, TUGGING AND DYEING MAKES IT MORE VULNERABLE," ADVISES DR. PAULA. SO, FOLLOWING DOCTOR'S ORDERS...

COLORING WILL ADD VOLUME. I'VE ALSO SET YOU UP WITH A STYLIST AND "THE FALL GUY."

YOU'RE SIX MONTHS PREGNANT. DON'T YOU HAVE ENOUGH TO DO?

THIS IS MORE IMPORTANT. IF YOU LOOK HEALTHY, YOU'LL FEEL HEALTHY. I LOVE YOU LIKE A SISTER AND I DON'T WANT YOU TO BE SICK.

BUT IF YOU *REALLY* WANT ME TO BE HAPPY, MAKE ME GO BLONDER.

WHILE UNDER THE DRYER...

I HAD BREAST CANCER AND DEVELOPED LYMPHEDEMA. DID ANYONE TELL YOU ABOUT IT?

A LITTLE BIT, HOW DID IT HAPPEN?

IF SHE HAD KNOWN ABOUT LYMPHEDEMA, IT MIGHT HAVE BEEN PREVENTED.

I TOUCHED HOT METAL AND MY ARM PLUMPED UP. NOW I HAVE TO WEAR THIS SLEEVE FOR THE REST OF MY LIFE TO AVOID ELEPHANTIASIS, LOSING MY ARM, OR DEATH...

THIS IS WHAT MADE ME CRY.

SHE HAD A DOUBLE MASTECTOMY AND TOTAL HAIR LOSS 3 YEARS AGO.

SO BE CAREFUL BECAUSE ANY CUT, STRAIN OR EXTREME TEMPERATURE CAN CAUSE IT... AND DON'T LET *ANYONE* CUT YOUR CUTICLES BECAUSE INFECTION CAN TRIGGER LYMPHEDEMA, TOO.

NEXT, BENOIT THE HAIRSTYLIST CUT 6 INCHES. 6 INCHES!

...AND YOU CAN PUT PIECES IN, LIKE PARIS HILTON. ALL HER HAIR IS FAKE.

AFTER MY CUT AND COLOR, I MET WITH NEIL, AKA "THE FALL GUY."

IF YOU ARE GOING TO LOSE 20% TO 50% OF YOUR HAIR, YOU CAN CONSIDER

A CLIP-ON,   A SEWN-IN,   OR A FUSION.

WHAT WOULD *I* NEED? ONLY TIME WOULD TELL...

AUGUST 11, THE DAY BEFORE CHEMO STARTS...

WHAT ARE YOU GOING TO WEAR? IT'S LIKE A PREMIERE.

I THINK IT'S MORE LIKE MY FIRST DAY OF SCHOOL.

I WENT FOR A SWIM TO PREPARE MYSELF PHYSICALLY...

72 LAPS = 1 MILE

THEN I WENT TO THE SHRINK TO PREPARE MYSELF MENTALLY...

YOU MUST BE FEELING DREAD WITH A CAPITAL "D."

DUH WITH A CAPITAL "D."

I MADE SURE I HAD ALL MY REPORTER SUPPLIES...
THIS TIME I WAS ON ASSIGNMENT FOR *GLAMOUR*.

TAPE RECORDERS SHOULD HAVE TAPES.

RadioShack

Mead

ACADEMIE Sketch Diary

I'M STILL VERY MANUAL

AT LEAST 1 THING IS DIGITAL, THAT'S AN IMPROVEMENT

THAT NIGHT, I WENT TO DA SILVANO AND GOT PREPARED SPIRITUALLY...

MARISA, BASTA!

I DIDN'T WANT TO BE JUST FILLED WITH DREAD

AND LATER GOT PREPARED EMOTIONALLY.

3:30 A.M. YOURS TRULY COULDN'T SLEEP...

NO DRINKING THE NIGHT BEFORE CHEMO!

OOPS! I ALREADY BLEW THAT ONE!

138

SO I WENT TO THE LAB FOR MY FIRST BLOOD TEST...

MIND IF I TAPE THIS? I'M DOING A PIECE FOR *GLAMOUR*.

RECORD

SURE HON, AND YOU CAN TAKE A PICTURE OF ME.

YVONNE "DOESN'T GIVE EVERYONE THAT PRIVILEGE."

WHEN'S YOUR BIRTHDAY?

MY BIRTHDAY? WHY ARE YOU ASKING, ARE YOU INTO ASTROLOGY?

WE ASK YOU THAT TO MAKE SURE YOU'RE YOU, AND YOU'RE GETTING THE RIGHT TREATMENT.

THAT'S OUR WAY OF DOUBLE-CHECKING.

DO YOU HAVE A PORT?

WHAT'S A PORT?

EXCUSE ME...

I HAVE A PORT, SEE?

A "MEDIPORT" IS INSERTED INTO PATIENTS WHO HAVE THIN VEINS, OR IF THEY'RE GETTING THE HEAVIER CHEMO

SPECIAL NEEDLES GO IN HERE

ACTUAL SIZE

I GUESS THEY DIDN'T THINK I NEEDED ONE.

MAKE A FIST FOR ME.

NEEDLE #6

THE "BLOOD-DRAWING NEEDLE"

SHE TOOK 2 VIALS.

OWW...

I TENSED MY FEET AS HARD AS I COULD.

THE ONLY THING THAT FELT OK WAS LOOKING AT MY SHOES.

ANY PAIN?

ONLY TO THE LEFT OF HER.

WAIT #2. THE RECEPTION AREA OF DR. PAULA KLEIN.

MARCHETTO!

WAIT TIME: 16 MINUTES

NEXT THEY SENT US TO AN EXAMINING ROOM.

Bridget Grimes Med. Ass.

THIS IS HOW THEY ABBREVIATE "MEDICAL ASSISTANT"?

BRIDGET TOOK MY TEMPERATURE, BLOOD PRESSURE, PULSE AND...

112 OVER 80, NORMAL.

WHEN IT COMES TO ANYTHING MEDICAL, THAT'S WHEN I WANT TO BE NORMAL!

WHAT? WHY DO I HAVE TO GET ON A SCALE?! *

* THEY NEED ALL THIS INFO SO THEY CAN MAKE THE APPROPRIATE DOSES.

IF I KNEW I HAD TO STEP ON A SCALE BEFORE EVERY TREATMENT, I WOULDN'T HAVE HAD LUNCH, DAMMIT!

YOU'RE GAINING WEIGHT.

THANKS FOR THE CARBS, MA!

WAIT #3: WE WAIT FOR DR. PAULA KLEIN AND NURSE SPECIALIST MARY ANN JULIANO.

MY (S)MOTHER TELLS ME SHE'S "DOING OK."

WAIT TIME: 6 MINUTES

WHY DO YOU HAVE A TAN?!

YOU HAVE TO BE REALLY CAREFUL. YOUR SKIN WILL BE EXTRA SENSITIVE TO THE SUN AND IT CAN BURN EASILY.

I TOLD HER TO STAY OUT OF THE SUN, BUT DID SHE LISTEN?!

SO WE'RE DOING LIGHT CHEMO SO YOU WON'T LOSE YOUR HAIR.

AND BECAUSE *YOU* SAID HEAVY CHEMO WASN'T NECESSARY.

THERE'S THAT TAPE RECORDER AGAIN.

IS IT OK, DOC?

IT'S FINE.

OK, LIGHT CHEMO, 8 TREATMENTS EVERY 3 WEEKS OVER 6 MONTHS BA, BA, BA...

WHOA!

...YOU'RE UP A FEW POUNDS FROM ITALY... YOU'RE GONNA GAIN *MORE WEIGHT!*

WHAT DO YOU MEAN I'M GONNA GAIN MORE WEIGHT?!?!

YOU CAN *GAIN* WEIGHT ON CHEMOTHERAPY PARTLY BECAUSE OF THE STEROIDS.

I KNOW I REALLY SHOULDN'T COMPLAIN, CONSIDERING I WON'T LOSE ALL MY HAIR.

YOU WON'T LOSE ALL YOUR HAIR.

ONE GIRL LOST HER HAIR, BUT HER HAIR WAS THIN TO BEGIN WITH.

MY HAIR IS THIN TO BEGIN WITH.

HER HAIR WAS *THINNING.*

MAYBE I SHOULD GET A WIG?

OK, HERE'S THE DRILL. DO YOUR LABS FIRST. WHILE THEY'RE BEING "COOKED" OR TESTED, YOUR BLOOD PRESSURE, PULSE AND TEMPERATURE ARE TAKEN AND YOU GET WEIGHED.

THEN WE GO OVER ANY SIDE EFFECTS YOU MAY HAVE.

NEXT WE WRITE THE ORDERS FOR THE DRUGS, SIGN THEM AND SEND THEM TO THE PHARMACY.

THE PHARMACY MIXES THE DRUGS, AND IT COULD TAKE AN HOUR.

THIS IS A LOT OF WAITING!

PLAN ON SPENDING HALF THE DAY HERE. IF YOUR LABS ARE OK, YOU'RE OK FOR CHEMO.

ME...OK FOR CHEMO...

MOM...?

How long are treatments?

How often are treatments?

How many treatments will I need?

How will I feel afterward?

Can I exercise?

Will I be tired?

What kind of exercise should I do?

Can I keep working?

Does each treatment get progressively worse?

Will I throw up?

Can I travel?

How nauseous will I be?

When will this ever end?

WAIT #4. THE CIRCULAR LOBBY OUTSIDE THE TREATMENT AREA, WHERE WE WAITED WHILE THE DRUGS WERE BEING MIXED.

THIS FEELS LIKE PURGATORY.

I FEEL LIKE I'M IN LIMBO.

WHAT A BEAUTIFUL DAY!

YOU AND SILVANO! I DON'T SEE WHAT'S SO *BELLA* ABOUT THIS LOUSY *GIORNATA!*

...AND WAITED...

MARCHETTO!

FINALMENTE!

WAIT TIME: 46 MINUTES

WAIT #5. THE TREATMENT AREA, WHERE YOU GET TREATED.

IS THE SEAT OK?

WHEN IT COMES TO CHEMO, IS THERE ANY GOOD SEAT IN THE HOUSE?

THERE ARE 3 STATIONS TO EVERY CHEMO BAY.

REAL IVY

EACH STATION IS EQUIPPED WITH A TV, PHONE AND A CHEMO CHAIR, WHICH IS LIKE A SOUPED UP LA-Z-BOY.

THE CHANNEL WITH THE BEST RECEPTION: "THE FOOD NETWORK," DAMMIT!

THIS GOES ALL THE WAY DOWN

SHELF

TRAY THAT FUNCTIONS AS A DESK WHERE I IMMEDIATELY SET UP SHOP

SHELF

THIS GOES ALL THE WAY UP

NEEDLE #7

THE CHEMO IV (#1 OF 8 TREATMENTS, EACH 3 WEEKS APART)

GOT IT.

=GASP!=

COLLEEN QUICKLY ASSEMBLES THE IV...

THE DRUGS ARE GIVEN THROUGH AN INTRAVENOUS CATHETER...

OWW! I REALLY DON'T WANT TO DO THIS.

BEING POSITIVE CAN HELP MAKE YOUR TREATMENT SUCCESSFUL.

ONE SEC, IT'S MY GLAMOUR EDITOR.

Lauren Callin[g]

HEY, HOW'S CANCER VIXEN?

SHE'S GETTING HER MATERIAL NOW.

MARY ANN, WHAT ARE THE OTHER SIDE EFFECTS NOW THAT I'M OFFICIALLY STUCK HERE?

THE SIDE EFFECTS OF CHEMOTHERAPY CAN BE CUMULATIVE. THERE'S RISK OF ANEMIA, CHANCES OF OSTEOPOROSIS, BONE MARROW SUPPRESSION, DIARRHEA, CONSTIPATION, IF YOU HAVE MORE THAN 4 LOOSE STOOLS YOU HAVE TO CALL ME. FATIGUE WILL HAPPEN IN WEEK 2, MOUTH SORES. WE ALREADY TOLD YOU ABOUT SUNBURN, AND WHENEVER YOU GO OUTSIDE YOU MUST WEAR SUNBLOCK, YOU MAY GET FUZZY ABOUT DETAILS IN GENERAL ...

IS THAT ALL ?!?

OH, AROUND THE 2ND OR 3RD TREATMENT, YOU MAY LOSE YOUR PERIOD.

IF I LOSE MY PERIOD, WHAT DOES THAT MEAN?

IT MEANS YOU'RE GOING THROUGH EARLY MENOPAUSE.

IF I'M GOING THROUGH EARLY MENOPAUSE, WHAT DOES THAT MEAN?

IN SOME CASES, INFERTILITY IS PERMANENT, IN SOME CASES IT'S TEMPORARY.

YOU SHOULD KNOW WE GAVE YOU A PREGNANCY TEST WHILE WE WERE DOING BLOOD WORK.

WHY?

IF YOU CONCEIVE WHILE RECEIVING CHEMO, IT MAY CAUSE BIRTH DEFECTS...

YOU DON'T HAVE TO TELL ME WHAT THAT MEANS...

...I WOULD HAVE TO ABORT.

MOM...?

149

HEY MOM!

UP HERE!

YOUR SON WANTED TO SAY GOODBYE.

MY TIME'S UP. I'M NOT HAPPENING IN THIS LIFETIME.

POOF!

I'M THE ONLY ONE YOU HAVE TIME FOR NOW, AND THE CLOCK'S TICK, TICK, TICKING...

ARE YOU OK? YOU LOOK UPSET.

WELL, I WAS JUST GIVEN SOME PRETTY TERRIBLE NEWS CONSIDERING I'M 43 AND IT'S ALREADY LATE FOR ME TO HAVE CHILDREN.

I'M SORRY.

ARE YOU OK?

I'M FINE.

NO SOY. SOY IS A PLANT ESTROGEN AND YOU HAD AN ESTROGEN RECEPTIVE TUMOR, WHICH MEANS THE TUMOR GREW IN THE PRESENCE OF ESTROGEN.

THANKS. I DON'T WANT TO GROW A NEW ONE.

YOU SHOULD TELL THAT TO YOUR FRIEND WHO RECOMMENDED THAT QUACK DOCTOR WHO TOLD YOU TO EAT SOY.

BASTARD!

OH, AND ONE LAST THING, NONE OF THOSE "IMMUNE BOOSTERS," NO JUICING, NO EXTRA VITAMINS, NO GREEN TEA AND NO ANTIOXIDANTS.

CHEMO WORKS BY ATTACKING THE QUICKER, MORE AGGRESSIVE RAPIDLY DIVIDING CANCER CELLS, AND THAT'S WHY HAIR LOSS IS A SIDE EFFECT. ALL CELLS NEED OXYGEN TO LIVE. THE ANTIOXIDANTS THAT WERE MEANT FOR NORMAL CELLS COULD BE FEEDING THE CANCER CELLS THE CHEMO IS TRYING TO KILL.

THE ENEMY IS ABOUT TO ATTACK!

RED ALERT!

FASTER! FASTER!

HURRY UP! HURRY UP! DIVIDE AND CONQUER!

I VANT TO BE A CLONE!

CANCER CELLS THRIVE IN CHAOS

SHAYNE SMALL, SVCCC NUTRITIONIST

A PLANT-BASED DIET IS THE BEST CANCER-REDUCING DIET.

TRY TO GET 9 SERVINGS OF FRUITS AND VEGETABLES; THE ONES WITH THE MOST COLOR HAVE THE MOST CANCER-FIGHTING NUTRIENTS.

HAVE BROWN RICE INSTEAD OF WHITE RICE. TRY TO FOCUS ON NONMEAT SOURCES OF PROTEIN; THE BEST ARE BEANS AND NUTS.

WHITE FLAKY FISH ARE ALSO LOW IN FAT.

I'M LEAN FROM ALL THAT SWIMMING.

IF YOU GRILL, CHARRING IS CARCINOGENIC, SO MARINATE MEATS IN VINEGAR; IT CUTS DOWN ON THE CARCINOGENS.

SHE GAVE ME A DIET BOOKLET ↙

AND LAST IS EVERYONE'S FAVORITE...

...LIMITING ALCOHOL!

I TOLD YOU!

JUST WHEN I THOUGHT IT COULDN'T GET ANY WORSE!

AFTER SHAYNE LEFT, I HAD A REACTION TO THE DECADRON, THE ANTINAUSEA STEROID I WAS GETTING THROUGH THE IV...

MY HAND IS FREEZING... AND IT'S NUMB...

AND WHAT'S CRAZY IS I'M SO HAPPY!

DECADRON COULD ALSO MAKE YOU FEEL HYPED FOR DAYS.

WRITE DOWN WHAT IT FEELS LIKE.

IT FEELS LIKE A TIDAL WAVE OF CRUSHED ICE...

...IS CRASHING THROUGH MY VEINS...

...AND THE FREEZING LIQUID IS FLOODING EVERY OUTLET IN MY SYSTEM...

BRRR!

"HERE HON, I GOT YOU A BLANKET."

"MOM, I GOT YOU SOMETHING..."

"IT'S A M.A.C LIPSTICK CALLED "FABBY.""

"OH, I LIKE IT."

AND NOW,

THE MOMENT I'VE BEEN WAITING FOR...

SARCASM DRIPPINGS ↓

"YOU WON'T FEEL A THING."

WAIT TIME FOR CHEMO: 38 MINUTES

"SO, HOW DO YOU MIX A CHEMO COCKTAIL?"

"YOU GET THE 3 DRUGS OF CMF, EACH 1 AT A TIME."

THE CHEMICALS WERE SO TOXIC, COLLEEN WORE HEAD-TO-TOE PLASTIC

FIRST IS METHOTREXATE, THE M OF CMF.

SHE PUSHED THIS INTO THE IV FOR 10 MINUTES.

METHOTREXATE BLOCKS AN ENZYME NEEDED BY A CELL TO LIVE.

NEXT IS FLUOROURACIL, THE F OF CMF.

AND SHE PUSHED THIS DRUG FOR ANOTHER 10 MINUTES.

BOTH FELT A LITTLE COOL GOING IN.

FLUOROURACIL PREVENTS THE GROWTH AND SPREAD OF CANCER CELLS.

CYTOXAN

LAST IS CYTOXAN, THE C OF CMF. YOU'LL BE ON THE "C" BAG FOR AN HOUR AND A HALF.

CYTOXAN DISRUPTS CANCER CELLS AND DESTROYS THEM.

WHILE ON THE "C" BAG...

BEEP!

CHEMO #1 DOWN, 7 MORE TO GO...

NURSE COLLEEN TOOK THE IV OUT.

TOTAL IV TIME: 2 HOURS, 22 MINUTES

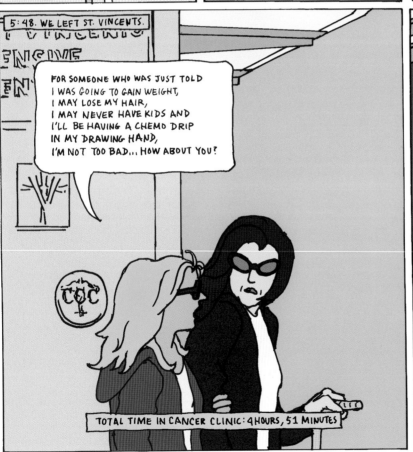

5:48. WE LEFT ST. VINCENTS.

FOR SOMEONE WHO WAS JUST TOLD I WAS GOING TO GAIN WEIGHT, I MAY LOSE MY HAIR, I MAY NEVER HAVE KIDS AND I'LL BE HAVING A CHEMO DRIP IN MY DRAWING HAND, I'M NOT TOO BAD... HOW ABOUT YOU?

TOTAL TIME IN CANCER CLINIC: 4 HOURS, 51 MINUTES

I'M WIPED OUT.

6:15. I CALLED SILVANO AFTER MY MOM DROVE ME HOME.

HI, MY LOVE, I FEEL GREAT, I'M JUST GOING TO TAKE A 20-MINUTE NAP.

10:30. I WOKE UP 4 HOURS LATER, BATHED IN MY OWN SWEAT.

MARISA, IT'S SILVANO. DO YOU FEEL LIKE COMING TO THE RESTAURANT?

ABSOLUTELY, I'LL BE RIGHT THERE.

SHOWING UP FOR MY MARRIAGE, MY CAREER AND THE PEOPLE WHO LOVE AND NEED ME WAS MY WAY OF FIGHTING.

QUICKLY I PULLED MYSELF TOGETHER, TRYING TO PUT THE HAPPY FACE ON...

WHERE IS MY LIPGLASS?

...AND RAN INTO THE RESTAURANT...

MARISA HA RICEVUTO CHEMOTERAPY OGGI, E—

— SILVANO.

ECCO MARISA.

CIAO, BABY, YOU LOOK FANTASTIC!

SILVANO WAS STILL WORKING, SO I MADE SMALL TALK WITH THE NEXT TABLE...

I JUST CAME BACK FROM ST. TROPEZ.

AND I WAS IN ST. BARTHS.

REALLY? I JUST CAME BACK FROM ST. VINCENTS.

ST. VINCENTS? I'VE NEVER BEEN TO THAT ISLAND.

HOW IS IT?

WELL, I JUST HAD TO GO.

I WAS TO GET TREATED EVERY 3 WEEKS, AND QUICKLY I FOUND OUT THERE WAS A RHYTHM TO IT,

WEEK 1. THE CHEMO HIGH. THE DAY AFTER, I WAS FLYING ON STEROIDS...

(NOT THINKING THAT IT WAS JUST 1 OF 21 "RECOVERY DAYS" UNTIL ROUND 2.)

IN FACT, I SWAM 74 LAPS...

...AND I COULD'VE KEPT GOING.

DAY 2. THE *GLAMOUR* GIRLS SENT ME A "YOU GO GIRL" BOUQUET.

Chemo Schmemo
xo

MAYBE THIS WASN'T THAT HARD?

DAY 3. I TOOK SOME EXTRA WORK FROM MY BFF ALEX.

WE'RE ON A TIGHT DEADLINE...

7 CARTOONS? YOU BET I CAN!

DAY 4. I STARTED TO COME DOWN...

HOW ABOUT WE GO TO BED...

...AND SLEEP.

DAY 5. WHILE ON DEADLINE FOR *GLAMOUR* AND *THE NEW YORKER* ...

WHY CAN'T I THINK OF ANYTHING?

DAY 6. MY DOCTORS TOLD ME THAT MY CELLS NEEDED TO REGENERATE, SO I TOOK IT EASY. AFTER ALL, I HAD TO SUPPORT MY TROOPS.

SLEEPING IN THE BUNKER BEFORE THE NEXT BATTLE

WEEK 3. THE CHEMO LEVELING OFF. JUST WHEN YOU'RE BACK TO YOUR OLD SELF...

BACK TO THOSE CRAZY CARTOONIST LUNCHES...

DIFFEE DOESN'T DRINK; WE'LL SPLIT HIS WINE.

I SHOULDN'T, BUT I WILL.

BACK TO A NAPLESS AFTERNOON...

CARTOONS FOR THE TENTS OF L.A. FASHION WEEK? I'D LOVE TO DO IT.

BACK TO THAT MILE-LONG SWIM 5 TIMES A WEEK...

DAY 17. I THREW A BACHELORETTE PARTY FOR MY FRIEND ANNE.

I'M TIRED. ARE YOU SURE YOU HAD CHEMO?

DAY 20. THE NIGHT BEFORE CHEMO #2, MY G)MOTHER CALLED...

MARISA, I HAVE A SORE THROAT AND YOU CAN'T BE AROUND ME.

THAT'S OK, MA. I'LL GO BY MYSELF. FEEL BETTER.

CHORTLE! CHORTLE! UGH GLUCK! UGH GLUCK!

THE GROSS-OUT-CLEARING-THE-THROAT-THING.

MUCH LATER...

IT'S 5:30 IN THE MORNING AND YOU NEVER CAME TO BED!

I'VE GOT TO FINISH THIS BEFORE TREATMENT.

1 P.M. THAT DAY...

FERN, I JUST E-MAILED YOU THE ART. WHEN DO THE TENTS GO UP?

TAXI!

DRIVER, CAN YOU TAKE ME TO 15TH BETWEEN 8TH AND 9TH AND STEP ON IT, PLEASE?

OWW... MY EARDRUM!

JUST WHEN YOU'RE BACK TO YOUR OLD SELF, IT'S CHEMO TIME ALL OVER AGAIN...

CHEMO #2. SEPTEMBER 2. 1:18. I WAS 18 MINUTES LATE.

SHOE: GIUSEPPE ZANOTTI FOR A HOT END-OF-THE-SUMMER DAY

WHILE I WAITED OUTSIDE THE LABS TO GET MY BLOOD WORK DONE...

ANYONE SITTING HERE?

JUST YOU TWO.

10 MINUTES LATER...

THEY CALLED ME FOR BLOODS. I'LL BE RIGHT BACK.

I WAS HERE FIRST! OOF! HOW LONG DO I HAVE TO WAIT?

SHUT UP. YOU'RE IN A CANCER TREATMENT CENTER!

SO WHAT! YOU SHUT UP!

MY WIFE DIDN'T GET OUT OF BED ALL WEEK...

...WHEN SHE'S NOT SLEEPING, SHE'S CRYING.

OH GOD!

≥ GASP! ≤

SMACK!

NOW HOW DO YOU FEEL?!

OUCH.

MARCHETTO!

YOU HAVE A LOT OF SPIRITUAL WORK TO DO!

I WAS TOO SHAKEN TO BE ANNOYED BY MY HIGHER SELF LOOKING DOWN ON ME.

HI. I WAS WAITING WITH YOU IN THE LOBBY.

HI AGAIN.

OH, I LOVE YOUR SHOES!

I NEVER SAW HER AGAIN. I PRAY AND HOPE SHE'S OK.

WHEN'S YOUR BIRTHDAY?

NEEDLE #8

THE BLOOD-DRAWING NEEDLE DREW 2 VIALS OF BLOOD...

PURPLE CAP = COMPREHENSIVE BLOOD COUNT (CBC COMP)

YELLOW CAP = TUMOR MARGINS

VIALS ARE THEN AGITATED TO DISTRIBUTE A WHITE SUBSTANCE WHICH STOPS THE BLOOD FROM CLOTTING BEFORE IT'S TESTED.

45 MINUTES LATER, AT THE CHEMO BAY...

WHEN'S YOUR BIRTHDAY?

THAT WAS MY CUE TO EXPECT ANOTHER WONDERFUL MOMENT, WHICH WAS...

YOU GAINED 2 POUNDS SINCE YOUR LAST TREATMENT.

WHAT? I DIDN'T EVEN HAVE LUNCH!

DAMN DIGITAL SCALE

AND I TOOK OFF MY SHOES, TOO.

NURSE MARY ANN PUT ME IN A PRIVATE ROOM. NO COMPLAINTS THERE.

YOUR WHITES ARE OK. READY FOR YOUR IV?

READY AS I'LL EVER BE!

WHEN'S YOUR BIRTHDAY?

SHE WAS A NEW NURSE. COLLEEN GOT PROMOTED. GOOD FOR HER. BAD FOR ME.

ANYTHING GOOD IN THE TABLOIDS?

FASHION DISASTERS, FEUDING STARLETS, SURFACING SEX TAPES TAKE MY FOCUS OFF THIS— CELEBRITIES ARE DOING SUCH GOOD THINGS FOR MANKIND AND THEY DON'T EVEN KNOW IT!

TAP! TAP!

OH, THERE'S YOUR VEIN.

NEEDLE #9

THE CHEMO IV (#2 OF 8)

FOR SOME REASON, THE DRUGS MADE ME HUNGRY. SO I MADE MY WAY TO THE KITCHEN...

TEA BAGS, HOT CHOCOLATE & SOUP MIX

HOT WATER, COLD WATER

COFFEE MACHINE

A VARIETY OF FLAVORED COFFEES

GRAHAM CRACKERS & PEANUT BUTTER CRACKERS

NUTRI-GRAIN BARS

THE IV MACHINE WAS ON WHEELS, SO I WAS MOBILE

I GRABBED A YOGURT

JUICES

SANDWICHES

BACK IN MY ROOM, I FELL ASLEEP ON THE C BAG WHEN...

THAT HEINOUS SMELL CAME FROM ME?!?

PFFT!

CHEMO FARTS

NOBODY, I MEAN NOBODY, TOLD ME ABOUT THEM.

BEFORE THE AIR CLEARED...

HI, DR. PAULA!

ENTER AT YOUR OWN RISK, DAMMIT!

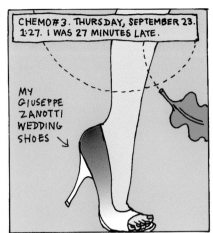

CHEMO #3. THURSDAY, SEPTEMBER 23. 1:27. I WAS 27 MINUTES LATE.

MY GIUSEPPE ZANOTTI WEDDING SHOES →

DO YOU HAVE A PORT?

NO, I HAVE AN ARM.

WHEN'S YOUR BIRTHDAY?

NEEDLE #10

THE BLOOD-DRAWING NEEDLE DREW 2 VIALS OF BLOOD.

I FEEL SORE-THROATISH.

YOU FEEL "SORE-THROATISH"?!

YOUR WHITES ARE LOW, WE'RE GOING TO TREAT YOU TODAY, BUT YOU HAVE TO GET A SHOT OF NEULASTA ON SATURDAY.

WHEN'S YOUR BIRTHDAY?

I GAINED 1 POUND?!

HAVEN'T LEARNED, HAVE YOU?

WHEN'S YOUR BIRTHDAY?

RATTLE! RATTLE! RATTLE!

NEEDLE #11

THE CHEMO IV (#3 OF 8)

WE HAD OUR FRIENDS ANNE AND PETER'S WEDDING PARTY THAT NIGHT IN CONNECTICUT...

DON'T KISS ME, I HAVE A SORE THROAT.

YOU DO? *

THE NEWLYWEDS

* REMINDER: ALWAYS CLUE YOUR MATE IN ON YOUR SURVIVAL TACTICS.

WE SAT WITH KIMBERLEY, MARION AND THEIR HUSBANDS, NIGEL AND BILL, AND HAD A GREAT TIME UNTIL...

HAHAHA? HAHA

SOMEONE TOLD A JOKE.

LAG TIME: 5 SECONDS

HA HA HA HAA...

MARISA, BABE... ARE YOU OK?

I CAN ALMOST DEAL WITH MY BODY FEELING SLUGGISH, BUT MY HEAD... I... MUST... HAVE... CHEMO BRAIN.

CHEMO BRAIN... WHAT'S THAT?

ANOTHER SIDE EFFECT. YOU FEEL LIKE YOUR GRAY MATTER TURNS TO MUSH.

COME ON, LET'S GO GET THE TRUFFLES.

OH, THAT'S WHAT I CAME OUT HERE FOR.

SHE HELD MY HAND BECAUSE I WAS A LITTLE WOBBLY.

ON THE WAY BACK TO THE CITY...

ARE YOU ANGRY WITH ME?

NO, I'M HAPPY WITH YOU. I'M JUST IN A LOT OF PAIN FROM THAT KILLER SHOT.

BUT I'M REALLY OK, OK?

OK.

THE LAST MONDAY IN SEPTEMBER, DR. PAULA AND NURSES MARY ANN AND COLLEEN JOINED ME FOR DINNER.

YOU REALLY *CAN'T* LOOK LIKE CRAP, I WON'T LET YOU!

THIS ISN'T REALITY.

THIS IS *MY* REALITY. THESE STICK FIGURES ARE ALWAYS HITTING ON MY HUSBAND.

THE BOTOXED BUTTLESS BLONDE BRIGADE

WHY ARE YOU SO INSECURE?

NURSE COLLEEN IS MY FAVORITE "NEEDLER!"

SILVANO COULD HAVE CHOSEN THE GIRL WITH THE BEST LEGS OR THE BEST BREASTS; INSTEAD HE MARRIED SOMEONE WITH BREAST CANCER, WHOSE MOST OUTSTANDING BODY PART IS HER NOSE.

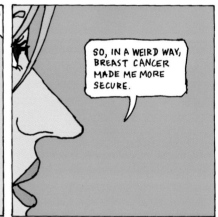

SO, IN A WEIRD WAY, BREAST CANCER MADE ME MORE SECURE.

SILVANO, CAN I HAVE A RIDE IN YOUR CAR?

SILVANO, TAKE ME DOWN TO YOUR WINE CELLAR?

'EY, I'M 'ERE WITH MY WIFE.

BUT I ADMIT IT'S A STRUGGLE WHEN 5'11" TWIGS MAKE ME FEEL LIKE A 5'2" STUMP.

THE NEXT TUESDAY I WENT TO *THE NEW YORKER*. AFTER MY DOSE OF REJECTION, I WALKED TO PERGOLA WITH ANOTHER GIRL CARTOONIST, CAROLITA JOHNSON.

DAMN MEDICAL MENOPAUSE! I AM A FURNACE!

HERE'S A CHINESE HERB THAT CAN HELP.

I LIKED CAROLITA IMMEDIATELY, BUT THE HERBS I HAD TO LOOK INTO.

HEY MARISA, HA HA... YOU'RE NOT THE ONLY GIRL AT LUNCH.

WILL YOU GUYS GROW UP? HOW OLD ARE YOU?

LATER, I RANG DR. GOLDSTEIN'S OFFICE. MARY ANN SAID IT WAS OK FOR ME TO GET A FLU SHOT.

WE ONLY GIVE FLU SHOTS TO PEOPLE WITH IMMUNITY PROBLEMS.

13TH ST

AS I WAS SAYING, IT'S A SPECIAL KIND OF CLUB.

SWIPE!

THE CANCER CARD

NEEDLE #15

THE FLU SHOT

THE NEXT DAY, I WENT TO SVCCC FOR SOME MORE CEMENT-IN-MY-VEINS, WHITE-BLOOD-CELL-SPURRING ACTION.

NEEDLE #16

THE NEULASTA SHOT

THIS IS EASY. I'M USED TO NEEDLES IN THE THIN SKIN OF MY HAND, NOT THE THICK SKIN OF MY ARM.

WHAT I WAS GETTING IMMUNE TO WAS PAIN.

YOU HAVE A SLIGHT TEMPERATURE. DON'T GO OUT IF YOU DON'T HAVE TO.

THAT'S TOO BAD. WHAT TIME WILL I SEE YOU AT MY SHOWER TONIGHT?

THE CANCER CARD
DECLINED

NEEDLESS TO SAY, I WENT TO SHARON'S SHOWER. SHE WAS THERE FOR ME, AND BESIDES...

...A NEW LIFE SHOULD BE CELEBRATED.

DAYS LATER, MY BFF ANNIE AND I WENT TO A BREAST CANCER PLAY.

...I WAS WITH MY SHRINK FOR YEARS, AND I JUST FELT I DIDN'T NEED HIM ANYMORE.

I'VE BEEN WITH MY SHRINK FOR 9 YEARS, AND I FEEL LIKE I NEED A NEW BOX OF TOOLS, BUT...

...HOW DO YOU BREAK UP WITH YOUR SHRINK?

HERE'S HOW. SILVANO AND I WENT TO L.A. FOR FASHION WEEK. MOST PEOPLE GO TO SEE THE SHOWS INSIDE THE TENT, BUT WE WENT TO SEE MY CARTOONS ON THE OUTSIDE OF THE TENT.

WE LEFT FOR LOS ANGELES ON SATURDAY,

AND TOOK THE RED-EYE BACK ON SUNDAY...

SPEAKING OF RED EYES, YOURS TRULY DIDN'T SLEEP A WINK...

7:45 A.M. I COLLAPSED INTO BED TO TAKE A NAP. MAYBE IT WAS THE WEEK 2 CHEMO LOW, OR MAYBE IT WAS THE RED-EYE, BUT I WOKE UP 12 HOURS LATER AND I ACCIDENTALLY STOOD UP MY SHRINK...

...WHO LEFT ME A VOICEMAIL...

MARISA, I THINK IT'S TIME WE STOP SEEING EACH OTHER.

I HAD A SLIP-UP ON CHEMO, AND SHE DUMPED ME.

LATER...

ARE YOU UPSET?

AHH...I'M NOT GOING TO WORRY ABOUT IT.

CHEMO 4. DAY 18. MY BFF BOB AND I WENT TO A FUND-RAISER FOR A BOOK CALLED *C101: BREAST CANCER BASICS FOR THE NEWLY DIAGNOSED.*

CAN'T DRINK, BABE. I'M COVERING THIS PARTY FOR MY *NY TIMES* COLUMN.

YOU'RE WRITING ABOUT CANCER FOR THE STYLES SECTION?

HOW STYLISH IS THAT PUCCI HEADWRAP? MAYBE I SHOULD'VE GOTTEN THE HEAVIER CHEMO.

STOP IT. YOU CAN'T JOKE ABOUT THAT!

A MILLISECOND LATER...

WHY ARE YOU HERE?

SAME REASON YOU'RE HERE. I'M GOING THROUGH CHEMO RIGHT NOW.

BUT YOU STILL HAVE YOUR HAIR!

I-I-I-I'M DOING THE LIGHTER CHEMO.

CHANGE YOUR DOCTOR! CHANGE YOUR PROTOCOL!

YOU HAVE TO BE AGGRESSIVE AND BOMB THE HELL OUT OF YOUR BODY...I DID!

MY MOTHER *DIED* FROM BREAST CANCER! IT'S CHRONIC AND IT DOES COME BACK!

ME, A MILLISECOND LATER...

GOD...PLEASE, *PLEASE* DON'T LET IT COME BACK.

AT THE KABBALAH CENTRE, I TOLD RUTHIE THE RABBI ABOUT BEING ASSAULTED AT THE C101 PARTY.

YOU BROUGHT THAT ON YOURSELF BY THAT ONE MOMENT OF DOUBT. YOU MUST STAY POSITIVE. YOU CAN'T EVEN JOKE ABOUT IT.

HOW BIG WAS THE TUMOR?

1.3 CENTIMETERS.

RUTHIE IS A KABBALAH TEACHER

1.3 CENTIMETERS IS THE SIZE OF A PEA...DON'T MAKE THIS ISSUE ANY BIGGER THAN IT IS.

I NAPPED FROM 6:30 TO 10:00, AND THEN I WAS WOKEN BY...

WE JUST GOT OUR SHIPMENT TODAY AND MARISA, I SAVED YOU THE MOST PERFECT WHITE TRUFFLE! WE ARE GOING TO 'AVE A FEAST!

I LOVE

THEY COME FROM ALBA, ITALY

NOVEMBER STARTS WHITE TRUFFLE SEASON

DOGS ARE BRED TO SNIFF THEM OUT OF THE GROUND

OUR BFFs RICHARD AND SESSA JOINED US FOR DINNER, THEY WERE THROWING OUR WEDDING PARTY.

THIS IS AMAZING.

AHH...CHE BEL PROFUMO!

UMM...WHERE SHOULD WE DO YOUR PARTY?

OHH... WHAT AN AROMA!

WHEN SUDDENLY...

SILVANO, GIVE ME YOUR CROSS.

FEASTUS INTERRUPTUS.

NO.

THE CROSS HAD SKULLS IN IT

I'M CATHOLIC. GIVE IT TO ME OR BUY ME ONE.

I'M WITH MY WIFE.

I DON'T CARE ABOUT YOUR WIFE. I WANT THAT CROSS.

NO.

THE EVENING WAS ALMOST RUINED...

UNBELIEVABLE.

DON'T LOOK AT 'ER, I'M NOT.

LATER THAT NIGHT...

PFFT!

PFFT!

WHITE TRUFFLES CAN MAKE ANYTHING SMELL GOOD.

WHAT A WONDERFUL WAY TO END A MEAL!

THE NEXT DAY, I TOLD RUTHIE THE RABBI ABOUT "THE CROSS GIRL."

WHY DO YOU ALWAYS LOOK AT CHAOS?

CHAOS LOOKS AT *ME*.

PHOTOSHOP.

PHOTOSHOP?!?!

YOU'RE AN ARTIST, YOU CAN CHANGE THE WAY CHAOS LOOKS...

PUT THEM IN PHOTOSHOP AND MAKE THEM INSIGNIFICANT.

THAT NIGHT...

SILVANO, CAN I SUCK ON YOUR CIGAR?

NO, AND THAT'S MY WIFE.

THEY'RE JEALOUS.

PAULA'S RIGHT. WHO CARES ABOUT THEM. THEY ALL LOOK THE SAME. THEY'RE FLAT ON THE FRONT AND FLAT ON THE BACK.

HMM...

Photoshop   File Edit Layer Select Filter View Window Help

Gradient Tool

Paint Bucket

Color   Swatche

DAY 10. MY ENERGY WAS THE LOWEST OF THE LOW...

CAPPUCCINO GETTING COLD!

AN HOUR LATER, I NUKED THAT CAPPUCCINO AND GOT TO WORK.

HEY LAUREN, I'M SENDING 12 PAGES OF *CANCER VIXEN*.

I THINK WE ONLY NEED 4.

NEW EXTENDED NAP TIME: 6-8:30 P.M.

MY NAPS INCREASED A HALF HOUR WITH EVERY CHEMO.

WEEK 3. THANKSGIVING. MY FAMILY AND I PLAYED SOUS CHEF TO THE MAESTRO WHO CONDUCTED THE HOLIDAY DINNER...

YUN, SHUCK THE OYSTERS.

DAVE, SHUCK THE SCALLOPS.

TONY, CUT THE BREAD.

DINA, CUT THE RADICCHIO.

MARISA, SLICE THE ARTICHOKES.

ANTHONY, TURN THE POTATOES.

VIOLETTA, DON'T PARBOIL THE BROCCOLI DI RAPE!

I AM THE BEST COOK IN NEW JERSEY, AND I ALWAYS PARBOIL BROCCOLI DI RAPE!

DO YOU WANT TO DO TINGS THE RIGHT WAY?

OK.

I AM IN SHOCK. NOBODY TELLS HER WHAT TO DO...

...AND LIVES.

IT WAS ONE OF THE MANY THINGS TO BE THANKFUL FOR.

LATER:

DELICIOSO!

FAVOLOSO!

I STILL THINK MY WAY IS BETTER!

THE DAY AFTER THANKSGIVING, I SWITCHED FROM SWIMMING TO RUNNING—IT BURNED MORE CALORIES.

X-MAS TREES

AFTER 2 MILES I WAS WINDED.

I COLLAPSED AFTER THAT CHEMO. AT 10:30 SILVANO CALLED...

MARISA, YOU DON'T 'AVE TO COME DOWN, I CAN SEND SOMETING UP...I MADE A NICE CAULIFLOWER AND BRUSSEL SPROUT SOUP, I KNOW 'OW YOU LOVE THEM! *

NO, I'LL COME OVER.

*CRUCIFEROUS VEGETABLES COMBAT CANCER.

WEDNESDAY, DECEMBER 1.

NEEDLE #21

THAT CREAKY-CEMENT-HARDENING-IN-MY-BONE-MARROW-NOT-SO-EASY-TO-MOVE-$3,500 SHOT OF NEULASTA ALMOST RUINED MY CHEMO HIGH...

NOTICE I SAID "ALMOST." THE NEXT DAY...

CONGRATULATIONS, BABY!

THANK YOU!

...I GOT AN OK FROM THE NEW YORKER.

I GOT MY ASS OUT 2 DAYS AFTER NEULASTA. NURSE MARY ANN SUGGESTED I WALK BECAUSE RUNNING MADE ME WINDED.

TOTAL MILES: 6

AND JUST WHEN YOU'RE (SORTA) BACK TO YOUR OLD SELF... IT'S CHEMO TIME ALL OVER AGAIN...

DAY 10. MY ENERGY HIT A NEW LOW ON THE DAY IT WAS USUALLY ITS LOWEST.

CAPPUCCINO IS COLD NOW!

AN HOUR AND A HALF LATER, I ADDED A SHOT OF ESPRESSO TO THAT CAPPUCCINO, NUKED IT AND WENT TO WORK.

I HAD TO FINISH THAT OK I GOT FROM THE NEW YORKER.

NEW EXTENDED NAP TIME: 6-9:30 P.M.

AND THEN, AFTER I PASSED THE HALFWAY POINT, JUST WHEN I COULD SEE THE LIGHT AT THE END OF THE TUNNEL, THE FINISH LINE, JUST WHEN I WAS ALMOST DONE WITH CHEMOTHERAPY, WHICH I'LL *NEVER REALLY KNOW* IF I NEEDED TO PREVENT A RECURRENCE OR NOT...

...A STORY APPEARED IN THE NEW YORK TIMES...

I READ A PAPER-LESS PAPER →

The New York Times
nytimes.com

December 11, 2004

Data Mounts on Avoiding Chemotherapy

By ANDREW POLLACK

New findings add to the evidence that genetic tests can help predict whether breast cancer will recur, giving valuable guidance to doctors and patients about whether potentially toxic chemotherapy will be useful or can safely be avoided, researchers said yesterday.

SO I ASKED DR. PAULA...

IT'S TOO LATE FOR YOU TO BE TESTED, YOU'RE ALMOST DONE WITH CHEMO.

OH WELL, I HOPE IT HELPS SOMEONE ELSE.

WEEK 3.

IT'S MY FAVORITE TIME OF THE YEAR...

I LOVE THE TREE...

I LOVE THE BIG SNOWFLAKES ON 57TH AND 5TH...

I LOVE THE DEPARTMENT STORE WINDOWS...

BUT THE DEPARTMENT STORES...

DAMN MEDICAL MENOPAUSE!

...CHRISTMAS SHOPPING AT BLOOMINGDALE'S. EXHAUSTING EVEN IF YOU'RE NOT ON CHEMO...

LYMPHEDEMA ALERT: I ONLY CARRY THINGS ON MY NON SURGERY SIDE.

YOU NEED THIS MORE THAN I DO. HAPPY HOLIDAYS!

WHO WAS MORE EMBARRASSED, THAT MAN FOR THINKING I WAS A BAG LADY, OR ME FOR LOOKING LIKE ONE?

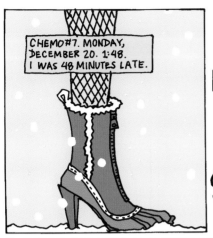

CHEMO#7. MONDAY, DECEMBER 20. 1:48. I WAS 48 MINUTES LATE.

WHEN'S YOUR BIRTHDAY?

NEEDLE # 22

THE BLOOD-DRAWING NEEDLE DREW 2 VIALS

WHEN'S YOUR BIRTHDAY?

GAINED 1 POUND

OH C'MON, IT'S ONCE A YEAR!

ABSOLUTELY *NOT*.

HAVE ANOTHER!

BASTA, MOM!

BUT I MADE THIS *ENTIRE* TIN FOR YOU!

MARISA!

MARY ANN, WE BROUGHT YOU SOME COOKIES.

OH, I'M ON A DIET.

BUT I'LL TAKE THEM ANYWAY.

✕✕✕✕! THERE GOES ALL MY HARD WORK!

ENJOY!

WHERE'S GINNY?

I DON'T KNOW WHERE GINNY IS.

DO YOU THINK SHE'S OK?

WHEN'S YOUR BIRTHDAY?

NEEDLE #23

THE CHEMO IV (#7 OF 8)

TAP! TAP!

TAP! TAP!

OK, THERE'S YOUR VEIN.

POP!

FIRST I WENT ON THE ANTINAUSEA WEIGHT-GAINING STEROIDS...

BRRR...

STILL NO GINNY.

THEN I GOT THE M PUSH

STILL NO GINNY.

THEN I GOT THE F PUSH.

I BROUGHT GINNY THE CORD OF ST. PHILOMENA.

I NEVER TOOK MINE OFF.

CYTOXAN

AND THEN I WENT ON THE C BAG.

HI GINNY, WE WERE LOOKING FOR YOU.

WE WERE LOOKING FOR YOU, TOO.

HI GINNY! HI JOHN!

I'VE BEEN PRAYING FOR YOU, DO YOU MIND IF I CONTINUE?

OH, PLEASE DO.

MY MOM TIED THE CORD OF ST. PHILOMENA ON HER WRIST.

THAT WAS THE LAST WE SAW OF PRETTY GINNY, WE PRAY AND HOPE SHE'S FINE.

OF COURSE I CONKED OUT ON THE C BAG...

BEEP!

CHEMO 7 DOWN 1 MORE TO GO

I CAN'T WAIT UNTIL THIS IS OVER.

WHY? YOU'RE NOT HAVING ANY FUN?

CHRISTMAS DAY. MY WHOLE FAMILY WENT DOWN TO MY **PARENTS'** HOUSE IN NEW JERSEY, WHERE THE MAESTRO ONCE AGAIN ORCHESTRATED A MASTERFUL MEAL.

DINA

JOHNNY

CARMINE

ANTHONY YUN DAVID

IT'S TALLER THAN HE IS!

'EY BREADMAN... IS THAT ENOUGH FOCACCIA FOR YOU?

DAD, THAT'S ENOUGH FOR A WEEK.

A 6 FOOT "SHEET"

BOB AND HIS NEW BOYFRIEND, IRA, DROVE IN FROM THE CITY... & SO DID OUR FRIENDS MIKE AND ILENE.

A GIFT FROM MY PARENTS

A PINK FUR HAT

I TOOK IT OFF BECAUSE IT WAS GIVING ME HOT FLASHES.

COUSINS MICHAEL, LINDA, VANNA AND GREAT AUNT DOLLY CAME OVER FROM DOWN THE STREET.

AFTER A SPECTACULAR FEAST OF FOIE GRAS ON FIG BREAD, OYSTERS, A SALAD OF RADICCHIO DI TREVISO, PUNTARELLE, FRESH SCALLOPS ON THE HALF SHELL, GRAPE TOMATOES AND LANGOUSTINES, LASAGNA, BRAISED ARTICHOKES AND PRIME RIB OF BEEF... IT WAS TIME FOR A CELEBRATION. THIS WASN'T JUST CHRISTMAS...

WHEN'S YOUR BIRTHDAY?

WERE YOU ACTUALLY *BORN* ON CHRISTMAS?

YEP. MY BIRTHDAY IS CHRISTMAS DAY.

I GAVE BIRTH RIGHT AFTER THE MEAL.

MY BABY SPENT 10 MONTHS IN THE WOMB.

LATE FOR HER OWN BIRTH.

I JUST WANTED TO SAY THAT I'M HAPPY YOU'RE ALL HERE...

↑ INK-STAINED HANDS, SOME THINGS NEVER CHANGE

I'M HAPPY TO BE HERE...

MY "SKULL WITH MICKEY MOUSE EARS" SWEATER- ← I WANTED TO LAUGH IN THE FACE OF DEATH

...I'M HAPPY TO BE ANYWHERE.

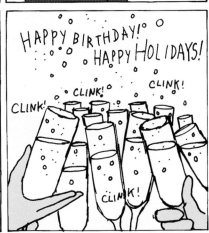

HAPPY BIRTHDAY! HAPPY *HOLIDAYS!*

CLINK! CLINK! CLINK! CLINK!

I'M SO HAPPY!

≥SOB! SOB! SOB!≥

WHAT'S YOUR MUDDER LIKE WHEN SHE'S MISERABLE?

AND THEN ME, THE FORMER MISS CONSUMED-WITH-GETTING-THE-RIGHT-BAG-INSTEAD-OF-GETTING-INSURANCE, THE GIRL WHO NEVER WANTED TO GROW UP, AT THAT MOMENT STOPPED DREADING EVERY SINGLE BIRTHDAY...

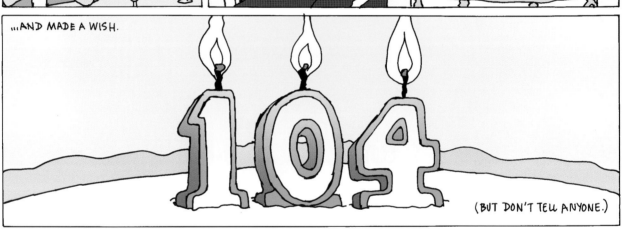

...AND MADE A WISH.

(BUT DON'T TELL ANYONE.)

I LOVE YOU, MARCHETTO.

I LOVE YOU TOO.

WHAT'S THAT? IS THAT A SMILE? IS BOB-A-SMILE-IS-WEAKNESS-MORRIS ACTUALLY SMILING?!?

HEY! THAT'S ENOUGH OUTTA YOU.

SHE BUSTED YOU, MR. MORRIS.

DAY 9 AFTER CHEMO. I WOKE UP FROM A NAP AT 10 P.M., FEELING DIZZY AND WEAK...

THAT'S 32 OUNCES OF POMEGRANATE JUICE ON A NEW OAK FLOOR.

CRASH!

SILVANO, I CAN'T DO IT. I CAN'T COME DOWN AT 10:30.

3 MINUTES LATER...

MARISA, ARE YOU OK?

I'M SORRY ABOUT THE FLOOR.

I'LL TAKE THAT, YOU LIE DOWN.

YOU'RE NOT GOING BACK TO THE RESTAURANT?

ALESSANDRO'S THERE. THAT'S WHAT MANAGERS ARE FOR.

DAY 10. MY LOW ENERGY DAY HIT A NEW LOW...

I WOKE UP 2 HOURS LATER, DRENCHED IN SWEAT AS USUAL.

CHEMO #8!!!
MONDAY,
JANUARY 13.

10:46. I CHECKED IN WITH ROY AT THE FRONT DESK 14 MINUTES EARLY.

TODAY'S YOUR LAST TREATMENT? ALLOW ME TO ESCORT YOU TO LABS.

BTW, MY LIPSTICK? "GIDDY," BY M.A.C.

WHEN'S YOUR BIRTHDAY?

?

TAP! TAP!

LET ME GUESS, YOU'RE A SCORPIO. SCORPION, STINGERS, NEEDLES... GET IT?

NEEDLE #24

THE BLOOD-DRAWING NEEDLE DREW 2 VIALS

WHEN'S YOUR BIRTHDAY?

YOU WANT ME TO TELL YOU?

YOU'RE SURE.

YEAH.

YEP.

YOU GAINED 2 POUNDS.

EH... YOU GAIN SOME, YOU LOSE SOME.

THEN I WENT TO SEE DR. PAULA...

NAUSEA? YES.
HOT FLASHES? YES.
NIGHT SWEATS? YES.
FATIGUE? YES.
DIARRHEA? YES.

HOW'S EVERYTHING ELSE?

I GOT NO COMPLAINTS.

STRESS BRINGS ON THE WORST HOT FLASHES!

THAT SHOULD DO IT.

I HOPE SO.

10 MINUTES LATER...

MY WHOLE ARM IS TOTALLY NUMB!

IT'S ICE COLD!

MY DAUGHTER CAN'T FEEL HER DRAWING HAND!

THIS IS GOING TO DESTROY HER...TAKE THAT THING OUT *NOW!*

WHAT'S THE MATTER?!

I'LL TAKE CARE OF IT!

IT WAS NURSES COLLEEN AND MARY ANN, WHO I SHOULD'VE CALLED AT THE BEGINNING.

YOU'RE GOING TO BE OK.

THIS IS YOUR LAST TREATMENT, SO WE CAN USE YOUR UPPER ARM.

NEEDLE # 27

THE CHEMO IV
(#10 OF 8 ✳ ✳ ✳ ✳ !!!)

AFTER ALL THE EXCITEMENT, I DIDN'T CRASH ON THE LAST SLEEP-INDUCING C BAG. HOW COULD I?

BEEP!

CHEMO #8 DONE. FINITO. TUTTO BASTA!

NEEDLE #28

A WEEK BEFORE I STARTED RADIATION, I WENT TO SVCCC TO GET TATTOOED.

YOU KNOW I'M KIDDING, RIGHT?

HERE'S MY TATTOO. TINY PERMANENT BLACK DOTS THAT FORM THE BLOCK WHERE I WAS GETTING RADIATED.

BE SURE TO MOISTURIZE AFTER EACH TREATMENT.

THEN I MET WITH RADIATION ONCOLOGIST DR. RESCIGNO...

THERE COULD STILL BE SOME LINGERING CANCER CELLS IN THE BREAST TISSUE THAT ARE TOO SMALL TO BE DETECTED. WE GIVE RADIATION TO PREVENT RECURRENCE IN THE BREAST, JUST TO BE SAFE.

SO, YOU'LL BE STARTING NEXT WEEK. 33 TREATMENTS, 5 DAYS A WEEK MONDAY THROUGH FRIDAY FOR 6½ WEEKS. ANY QUESTIONS?

YEP. I'M DOING FINAL ART ON MY GLAMOUR PIECE. ARE YOU SURE YOU DON'T WANT TO BE IN IT?

FEBRUARY 16, THE NIGHT BEFORE I STARTED TREATMENT...

GOD' NEWS, BABY! I GOT THE CAR SHOWROOM! WE'RE 'AVING OUR WEDDING PARTY MARCH 9. BUT DO YOU REALLY WANT TO DO IT IN THE MIDDLE OF RADIATION?

WHY CELEBRATE TOMORROW WHAT YOU CAN CELEBRATE TODAY?

THE NEXT DAY...

HEY SESSA, WE'RE DOING THE PARTY. SO, I'LL GET YOU OUR LIST OF ADDRESSES SO YOU CAN SEND OUT THE INVITES.

SURE, WHEN'S THE PARTY?

3 WEEKS? YOU BETTER GET ME SOME NUMBERS AND I'LL START DIALING. WHAT ARE YOU DOING NOW?

OH, I'M OFF TO GET NUKED.

194

AND NOW, IT'S TIME
TO ENTER A NEW PHASE
OF TREATMENT,
YOU KNOW...
"JUST TO BE SAFE"...

TURN PAGE TO OPEN DOOR AND DO IT 33 TIMES

MARCH 8. 10:15 A.M.

MARISA, IT'S LAUREN. WE HAVE A FEW MORE REVISIONS BEFORE *CANCER VIXEN* GOES TO PRINT, BUT ON A LIGHTER NOTE... WHAT ARE YOU WEARING TO YOUR PARTY TOMORROW?

I HAVEN'T GOTTEN A DRESS YET, I'VE BEEN TOO BUSY REVISING AND RADIATING.

OOPS. REMEMBER THE FASHIONISTA WHO WAS IN DENIAL ABOUT HER HEALTH?

GET OFF THE PHONE WITH ME AND GO FIND A DRESS RIGHT NOW!

SO I GOT MANICURED...

BROW-WAXED...

BEAMED...

BLONDED...

(NOW THAT I WAS OFF CHEMO, I WAS GOOD TO GO.)

AND OUTFITTED...

THIS DRESS IS TOO LOW...   THIS DRESS IS TOO TIGHT...   ...THIS DRESS IS JUST RIGHT.

RADIATION BURN

DAWN, COOL STYLIST AT McQUEEN

HOW ABOUT THIS?

WE COULD HAVE IT ALTERED, WHEN'S YOUR WEDDING PARTY?

YOUR WEDDING PARTY IS TOMORROW NIGHT?!

YOU'RE GIVING ME A HEART ATTACK!

198

MY LAST DOSE OF RADIATION...

I REMEMBER WISHING IT WOULD END ALREADY

FAST.

THEN I THOUGHT ABOUT THE FINITE LENGTH OF LIFE... AND HOW WE'RE ONLY HERE FOR A SHORT TIME...

WHY WOULD I WANT EVEN A MOMENT TO DISAPPEAR?

CLICK!

AND THAT WAS NUMBER 33!

AFTER PLEASE GOD MY FINAL BLAST, DR. RESCIGNO WANTED TO SEE ME.

WHY DIDN'T YOU PUT ME IN THIS?!

GLAMOUR

CANCER VIXEN HAD JUST COME OUT.

I ASKED YOU A MILLION TIMES AND YOU SAID NO. NO. NO.

WELL...

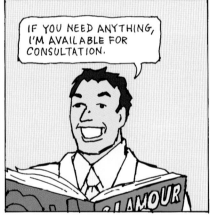

IF YOU NEED ANYTHING, I'M AVAILABLE FOR CONSULTATION.

GLAMOUR

SO I SAID MY GOOD-BYES TO ALL THE RADIATION TECHNICIANS...

BYE!

SO LONG!

CIAO!

I HOPE I NEVER HAVE TO SEE YOU AGAIN!

BUT I'LL ALWAYS LOOK FOR YOUR CARTOONS!

IF I WANTED TO SEE MY CARTOONS IN *THE NEW YORKER*, I'D HAVE TO BE SEEN BY *THE NEW YORKER*...

COME ON, COME TO *THE NEW YORKER* PARTY WITH ME.

CARTOONISTS HATE BEING AWAY FROM THEIR DRAWING BOARDS.

I DON'T KNOW.

OH COME ON, I HAVE YOUR BIRTHDAY GIFT AND IT'S APRIL ALREADY.

SAM DOESN'T HAVE A CELL PHONE AND HE DOESN'T HAVE E-MAIL.

SHOW YOUR FACE AND WE'LL HAVE SOME YUCKS.

HE ALSO DRAWS WITH A RAPIDOGRAPH THAT'S BEEN DISCONTINUED.

AN ORIGINAL "S. GROSS"!

COPYRIGHT 1974 S. GROSS

I LOVE IT!

I KNEW YOU WOULD, KIDDO. C'MON, LET'S GET SOME BOOZE.

REMEMBER WHAT HAPPENED 3 YEARS AGO WITH YOUR PAL?

RIVAL CARTOON GIRL?

IT'S ABOUT TO HAPPEN AGAIN.

NO IT'S NOT...

...I'M NOT THE SAME PETTY PERSON I WAS BEFORE CANCER...

...I'M COMING FROM A HIGHER PLACE.

OH YEAH?

HELLO, HOW ARE YOU?

HOW YA DOING?

IF I COULD FORGIVE HER, AND SHE COULD FORGIVE ME, MAYBE THERE WAS HOPE IN THE WORLD?

THE NEXT WEEK, I SPOKE TO RUTHIE THE RABBI...

WHEN SOMEONE ELSE'S GARBAGE MAKES US CRAZY, IT'S BECAUSE WE'RE MAKING SOMEONE ELSE CRAZY WITH THE SAME GARBAGE. LOOK AT THOSE DESPERATE WOMEN; WHEN THEY BOTHERED YOU THE MOST, YOU WERE THE MOST DESPERATE.

BUT THOSE WOMEN—

—STOP.

WHEN YOU POINT A FINGER AT SOMEONE...

RUTHIE ALWAYS HAS RED NAILS

...THERE ARE 3 FINGERS POINTING BACK AT YOU.

MEANWHILE, AT DA SILVANO...

I'M IN REMISSION.

I HAD BOTH BREASTS REMOVED.

DON'T CARRY YOUR BAG ON YOUR SURGERY SIDE. I HAVE LYMPHEDEMA.

YOUR HUSBAND SAID YOU WOULD TALK ABOUT IT.

SURE. JUST DON'T ASK ME "WHEN'S YOUR BIRTHDAY?"

AND AS I LOOKED AROUND ME, I SAW LESS AND LESS OF THE EVIL EYE.

ARE YOU OK? TAKE CARE HOW ARE YOU FEELING?

MAYBE I WASN'T LOOKING FOR IT, OR MAYBE I WASN'T GIVING IT. (AS MUCH)

THE EYES ARE THE REFLECTORS OF THE SOUL.

I NOTICE WHEN YOU GIVE PEOPLE "THE GOOD EYE," IT'S HARD HAVING A HATEFUL THOUGHT.

APRIL 28. I HAD A FOLLOW-UP WITH DR. PAULA AND NURSE MARY ANN.

WE'RE PUTTING YOU ON TAMOXIFEN. IT BLOCKS THE ESTROGEN IN THE BREASTS AND SLOWS THE GROWTH OF CANCER CELLS.

WHILE YOU'RE ON IT, YOU SHOULDN'T CONCEIVE.

HOW LONG WILL I BE ON IT?

FIVE YEARS.

44 + 5 = 49.

MOM....?

I'M SO SORRY... I THOUGHT I HAD ALL THE TIME IN THE WORLD, WHEN ALL I HAD WAS THE BLINK OF AN EYE.

GOOD-BYE,

POOF!

MOM...?

I'M SO SORRY,

I ALWAYS THOUGHT YOU'D HAVE A LITTLE GIRL.

⧽ SNIFF! ⧼

ARE YOU OK?

I'M FINE.

NEXT STEPS: ANNUAL OPHTHALMOLOGIST TO CHECK FOR OCULAR TOXICITY, ANNUAL GYNECOLOGIST TO LOOK AT YOUR OVARIES AND UTERUS, 1,200 MG OF CALCIUM AND 400 IU OF VITAMIN D FOR BASELINE BONE DENSITY AND SEE ME EVERY FOUR MONTHS, ALRIGHT?

THAT NIGHT AT DA SILVANO...

SILVANO, IT'S OFFICIAL. I'LL NEVER BE ABLE TO HAVE CHILDREN...

I'M SO 'APPY YOU'RE GOING TO BE OK.

...AND I'VE ALWAYS WANTED TO HAVE A GIRL, SO I'M SO THANKFUL THAT LEYLA IS THE GREATEST STEPDAUGHTER IN THE WORLD.

MAY 15. "D. DAY." DIAGNOSIS DAY, ONE YEAR LATER. SILVANO PLANNED A BIG SURPRISE FOR ME.

FATHER JAKE! MARISA!

FATHER PETER JACOBS IS A PRIEST IN THE VATICAN, AND OUR BFF.

BEFORE LUNCH, HE SAID A PRAYER FOR ME...

...NEL NOME DEL PADRE E DEL FIGLIO E DELLO SPIRITO SANTO. AMEN.

AND THEN...

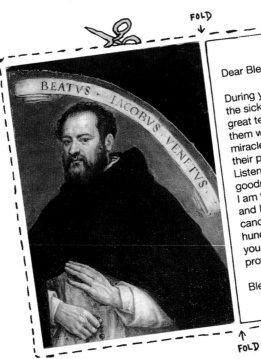

BEATVS · IACOBVS · VENETVS ·

Dear Blessed Iacobus,

During your lifetime you received the sick and the suffering with great tenderness, and you comforted them with words and performed miracles that helped them overcome their pain.
Listen to my prayer, and in your goodness, please help me. I am trying to be patient in adversity, and I pray to be protected from this cancer, for which people for hundreds of years have prayed to you and invoked your special protection.

Blessed Iacobus, pray for me.

FOLD

FOLD

TRANSLATED BY FATHER JAKE

FATHER JACOBS GAVE ME THIS HOLY CARD. BLESSED IACOBUS WAS BORN IN VENICE IN 1231, WHERE HIS RELICS ARE CONSERVED IN THE BASILICA OF SAINTS JOHN AND PAUL. HE IS PRAYED TO FOR HELP TO CURE CANCER. FATHER JAKE HAS WITNESSED 4 DRAMATIC MIRACLES.

SO, WHAT SHOULD WE EAT?

I WISH IT WERE THAT EASY.

TODAY I'M CANCER FREE, BUT WHENEVER I HAVE A MAMMOGRAM...

MARISA?

YOU CAN CHANGE OUT OF YOUR GOWN.

OK.

...THERE WILL ALWAYS BE A SECOND WHERE I LOSE MY BREATH.

REMEMBER THAT BREAST CANCER-SKIN CANCER LINK?

I NEED TO BIOPSY THAT MOLE ON YOUR BACK.

NEEDLE #29

A BAD SIGN?

DR. STROBER FOUND A MELANOMA, BUT ONCE AGAIN, I WAS LUCKY. IT WAS IN THE EARLY STAGE OF "IN SITU."

HAVING CANCER MANIFEST IN YOUR BODY NOT ONCE BUT TWICE IS LIKE LIVING ON HIGH ALERT.

IF THERE ARE ANY SLEEPING CANCER CELLS, I HOPE THEY REMAIN DORMANT.

GOD FORBID, IF I DO HAVE A RECURRENCE...

YOU'RE IN FOR THE FIGHT OF YOUR LIFE.

DITTO.

BASICALLY, I STILL HAVE A LOT OF SPIRITUAL WORK,

SMACK!

OUCH!

GIVE THE GOOD EYE!

A LOT OF PHYSICAL WORK,

YEAH, I'M ON A DIET, BUT I'M NOT DOING IT TO HAVE THE "IT" BODY.

EXERCISE AND A LOW BODY WEIGHT CAN HELP PREVENT RECURRENCE.

AND A LOT OF EMOTIONAL WORK TO DO.

I STILL KILL MYSELF ON DEADLINES...

...BUT STAYING ALIVE IS A BIGGER JOB AND IT'S NOT LIKE I'M OFF AT 5:00.

ANSWER:

IT ADDS UP TO AN EXPERIENCE
THAT HAS CHANGED ME FOREVER...

JUNE 14. WE WERE COMING BACK FROM THE MONTREAL GRAND PRIX. IT WAS OUR 1-YEAR ANNIVERSARY WEEKEND...

THIS IS THE WORST STORM I 'AVE EVER SEEN.

EXCEPT FOR IN A MOVIE.

I CAN'T SEE ANYTING.

I 'AVE TO PULL OVER.

THERE'S A PARTY FOR 60 PEOPLE AT THE RESTAURANT TONIGHT...

MOTOROLA

Emergency Use Only

...AND I CAN'T DIAL OUT.

WE'RE IN A BLACK 'OLE.

THANK YOU TO MY SUPPORT GROUP OF FAMILY AND FRIENDS.

THIS BOOK WOULD NOT EXIST WITHOUT THE CONTINUAL ENCOURAGEMENT OF CINDI LEIVE AND LAUREN SMITH BRODY OF *GLAMOUR*; MY AGENT, ELIZABETH SHEINKMAN; MY EDITOR/SISTER ROBIN DESSER, DIANA TEJERINA, ANDY HUGHES, PAUL BOGAARDS AND SONNY MEHTA OF KNOPF; AND CRAIG GERING AND SALLY WILLCOX AT CAA.

I WOULD ALSO LIKE TO ACKNOWLEDGE THOSE WHO WILL BATTLE, WHO ARE BATTLING, AND WHO HAVE BATTLED NOT JUST BREAST CANCER, BUT ALL CANCERS.

I PRAY FOR A CURE, AND LOOK FORWARD TO THE DAY WE ARE ALL CANCER-FREE.

IN MEMORY OF JIM MARSHALL AND LORNA CLARKE.

A NOTE ABOUT THE AUTHOR

MARISA ACOCELLA MARCHETTO LIVES IN NEW YORK CITY AND IS A CARTOONIST FOR *THE NEW YORKER* AND *GLAMOUR*.
HER WORK HAS APPEARED IN *THE NEW YORK TIMES* AND *MODERN BRIDE*, AMONG OTHER PUBLICATIONS.
SHE IS ALSO THE AUTHOR OF *JUST WHO THE HELL IS SHE, ANYWAY?*

GRATEFUL THANKS FOR THE SUPERB COLOR WORK BY JASON ZAMAJTUK AND DENNIS BICKSLER AND THE TEAM
AT NORTH MARKET STREET GRAPHICS.